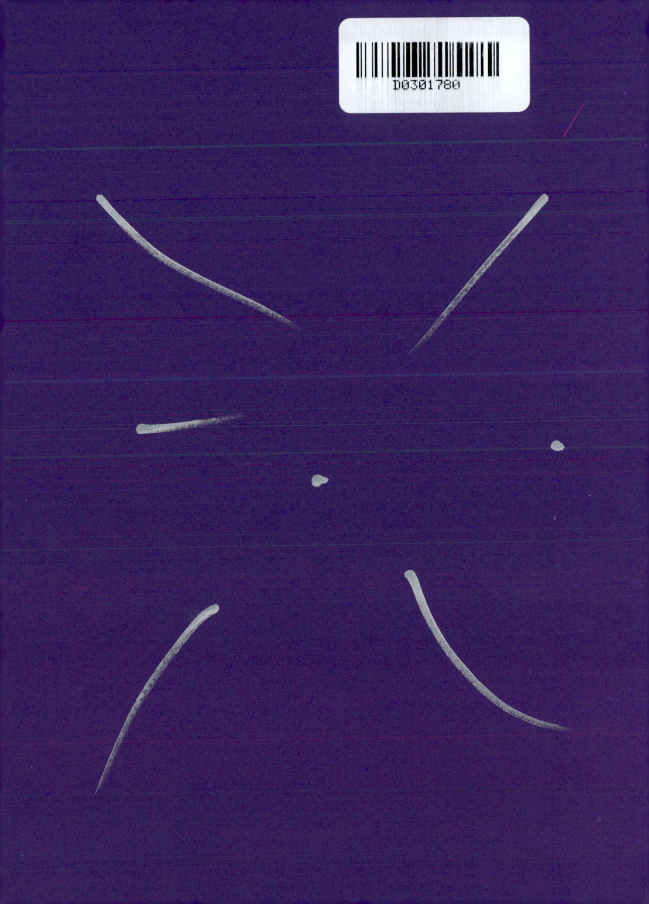

Complex Primary
Total Hip Replacement

18th Sept 2018.

Dear Rob,

With Best Wishes.

Manishyu

(SANJIV)
C.

Complex Primary Total Hip Replacement

SKS MARYA MS DNB MCh (UK) FICS
Vice Chairman
Max Healthcare
Chairman and Chief Surgeon
Max Institute of Orthopedics and Joint Replacement Surgery
New Delhi, India
sksmarya@yahoo.co.in

Foreword
Thomas P Sculco

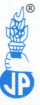

JAYPEE BROTHERS MEDICAL PUBLISHERS (P) LTD

New Delhi • Panama City • London • Dhaka • Kathmandu

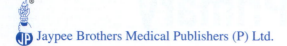
Jaypee Brothers Medical Publishers (P) Ltd.

Headquarter

Jaypee Brothers Medical Publishers (P) Ltd
4838/24, Ansari Road, Daryaganj
New Delhi 110 002, India
Phone: +91-11-43574357
Fax: +91-11-43574314
Email: jaypee@jaypeebrothers.com

Overseas Offices

J.P. Medical Ltd
83 Victoria Street, London
SW1H 0HW (UK)
Phone: +44-2031708910
Fax: +02-03-0086180
Email: info@jpmedpub.com

Jaypee Brothers Medical Publishers (P) Ltd
17/1-B Babar Road, Block-B, Shaymali
Mohammadpur, Dhaka-1207
Bangladesh
Mobile: +08801912003485
Email: jaypeedhaka@gmail.com

Jaypee-Highlights Medical Publishers Inc.
City of Knowledge, Bld. 237, Clayton
Panama City, Panama
Phone: +507-301-0496
Fax: +507-301-0499
Email: cservice@jphmedical.com

Jaypee Brothers Medical Publishers (P) Ltd
Shorakhute, Kathmandu
Nepal
Phone: +00977-9841528578
Email: jaypee.nepal@gmail.com

Website: www.jaypeebrothers.com
Website: www.jaypeedigital.com

Inquiries for bulk sales may be solicited at: jaypee@jaypeebrothers.com

This book has been published in good faith that the contents provided by the contributors contained herein are original, and is intended for educational purposes only. While every effort is made to ensure a accuracy of information, the publisher and the editor specifically disclaim any damage, liability, or loss incurred, directly or indirectly, from the use or application of any of the contents of this work. If not specifically stated, all figures and tables are courtesy of the editor. Where appropriate, the readers should consult with a specialist or contact the manufacturer of the drug or device.

Complex Primary Total Hip Replacement

First Edition: 2012

ISBN 978-93-5025-584-1

Printed at: Ajanta Offset & Packagings Ltd., New Delhi

Dedicated to

My forefathers

My great-grandfather
Dr Balmukand Singh Marya

My grandfather
Dr Raghunath Singh Marya

My father
Dr Sarwan Kumar Singh Marya

*All these surgeons made sure that I would be no good
for anything but surgery*

Contributors

Albert D'Souza
Attending Consultant Orthopedics
Max Institute of Orthopedics and Joint Replacement
Max Superspeciality Hospital
New Delhi, India

Anil Mehtani
Professor and Head
Department of Orthopedics
Lady Harding Medical College
New Delhi, India

Arvind Arora
Lecturer
King Edward VII Memorial Hospital
and GS Medical College
Mumbai, Maharashtra, India

Ashok Kumar
Department of Orthopedics
All India Institute of Medical Sciences
New Delhi, India

Chandeep Singh
Consultant Orthopedics
Max Institute of Orthopedics and Joint Replacement
Max Superspecialty Hospital
New Delhi, India

C Thakkar
Arthroplasty Surgeon
Breach Candy and Leelawati Hospital
Mumbai, Maharashtra, India

Henry Budd
Specialist Registrar
Cambridge Orthopedic Training Program
Cambridge, United Kingdom

HR Jhunjhunwala
Senior Consultant Orthopedic Surgeon
Postgraduate Institute of Medical Sciences
Bombay Hospital,
Mumbai, Maharashtra, India

JA Pachore
Director of Hip Surgery
Shalby Hospitals
Ahmedabad, Gujarat, India

Kamal Deep
Consultant Orthopedic Surgeon
Golden Jubilee National Hospital
and Ross Hall Hospital
Glasgow, United Kingdom

Mandeep S Dhillon
Professor and Head
Department of Orthopedics, PGIMER
Chandigarh, India

P Suryanarayan
Consultant, Joint Replacement Surgeon
Apollo Hospitals,
Chennai, Tamil Nadu
India

Rajesh Bawari
Senior Consultant Orthopedics
Max Institute of Orthopedics and Joint Replacement
Max Superspecialty Hospital
New Delhi, India

Rajesh Malhotra
Professor of Orthopedics
All India Institute of Medical Sciences
New Delhi, India

Rajiv Thukral
Senior Consultant Orthopedics
Max Institute of Orthopedics and Joint Replacement
Max Superspecialty Hospital
New Delhi, India

Sachin G Gujarathi
Junior Arthroplasty Consultant
Shalby Hospitals
Ahmedabad, Gujarat
India

Sarvdeep S Dhatt
Assistant Professor
Department of Orthopedics, PGIMER
Chandigarh, India

Shah Alam Khan
Additional Professor
Department of Orthopedics
All India Institute of Medical Sciences
New Delhi, India

Shishir Rastogi
Professor of Orthopedics
All India Institute of Medical Sciences
New Delhi, India

Shitij Kacker
Attending Consultant Orthopedics
Max Institute of Orthopedics
and Joint Replacement
Max Superspecialty Hospital
New Delhi, India

Shivan Marya
SHO Orthopedics
Queen's Hospital Romford
London, United Kingdom

SKS Marya
Vice Chairman—Max Healthcare
Chairman and Chief Surgeon
Max Institute of Orthopedics
and Joint Replacement Surgery
New Delhi, India

Sumeet Rastogi
Consultant Orthopedics
Max Institute of Orthopedics and Joint Replacement
Max Superspecialty Hospital
New Delhi, India

SV Vaidya
Professor and Unit Head
King Edward VII Memorial Hospital
and GS Medical College
Mumbai, Maharashtra, India
Joint Replacement Surgeon
Cumballa Hill Hospital
Mumbai, Maharashtra, India

Vijay C Bose
Consultant Orthopedic Surgeon
Apollo Specialty Hospital
Chennai, Tamil Nadu, India

Vikas Khanduja
Consultant Orthopedic Surgeon
Addenbrooke's-Cambridge University Hospital
Cambridge CB2 2QQ, United Kingdom

Vikram I Shah
Chairman and Managing Director
Shalby Hospitals
Ahmedabad, Gujarat, India

Yatinder Kharbanda
Senior Consultant Orthopedics
Indraprastha Apollo Hospital
New Delhi, India

Foreword

Total hip replacement is a highly successful surgical procedure which has helped countless patients returns to excellent function without hip pain. It demands accurate surgical technique and management to effect a total hip arthroplasty which will be durable and long lived. Attention to soft tissue as well as bony reconstruction is necessary to produce a biomechanically functional result. In the more complex primary hip replacement these techniques become more challenging and catastrophic results may occur if comprehensive and careful surgical techniques are not performed. Patients 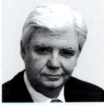 with previous fractures about the hip, severe hip dysplasia, tumors involving the hip and severe ankylosis all require advanced surgical principles and implant selection. SKS Marya has produced a textbook dealing with these more complex problems which thoroughly covers all aspects of the complex primary hip requiring arthroplasty surgery. Each chapter provides the reader with a complete review of the pathological problems to be encountered, a rationale for preoperative planning and correction of bony and soft tissue abnormality and discussion of implant options.

The text is comprehensive and each chapter is written in a clear and outstanding fashion. The illustrations are beautifully presented and extremely helpful to the reader. The most complex primary hip problems are all present and those unfamiliar with tuberculosis of the hip will find a very interesting and informative chapter on this topic. The author Marya has selected to contribute chapters are the most experienced and knowledgeable about hip surgery. This text fills a very important void in dealing with the complex hip patient and all information regarding technique and management of these difficult cases are here in this wonderful book. Dr Marya is to be congratulated on adding this most important textbook to the orthopedic literature and I congratulate him on an outstanding and very readable text. It will be a book which will teach and inform countless hip surgeons and will be a great addition to any library in orthopedic surgery.

Thomas P Sculco
Surgeon-in-Chief
Hospital for Special Surgery
New York, USA

Preface

If primary hip replacement is akin to driving on Mumbai-Pune highway, *Complex Primary Total Hip Replacement* is like driving on a steep mountainous road. Both need basic driving skills, licence to drive and caution while driving. However, driving in the hills carries a certain degree of risk and needs additional precautions besides being aware of small facts like "not to overtake on turns".

The idea to put this volume together has been nagging me for a long period of time. It would get activated every now and then when I would encounter difficulty negotiating a difficult primary hip replacement. I would then think of sharing my experience with some of my younger colleagues. More often than not a verbal discussion would ensue and the matter would end there. Finally we decided that for larger benefit we should document our collective experience and hence the birth of this book.

The volume opens with convenient exposures in inconvenient situations and concludes with evaluation of patients with persistent pain following complex primary hip replacements. It also covers a spectrum from excision hip arthroplasty to computer assisted hip replacement. We have tried to analyze difficulty in performing such surgery in situations such as avascular necrosis of femoral head, fractures, failed fixations, tumors and protrusion. In addition the authors have expressed their views in tackling the challenges in osteoporotic situations, ankylosing spondylitis, rheumatoid arthritis and infections. We have rounded off with topics dealing with hip replacements in dysplastic hips, proximal femoral deformities and an overview of total hip replacement in patients with neuromuscular abnormalities.

A galaxy of experienced and enthusiastic surgeons with varying interests were roped in to pen down their advises. An attempt has been made to cover a considerable width of complex primary situations. I would hope that the readers will synthesize their experience with those of the authors and enjoy performing more complex primary hip replacements with minimal difficulty and maximum pleasure.

SKS Marya
President, Indian Orthopedic Association, 2013
President, Indian Arthroplasty Association
President, Indian Society of Hip and Knee Surgeons
Chairman, Knee Arthroplasty SICOT
(International Society of Orthopedic Surgery and Traumatology)
President, India and SAARC: International Congress of Joint Reconstruction
Permanent Board Member, Asia Pacific Arthroplasty Society
sksmarya@yahoo.co.in

Acknowledgments

This book would be half complete and not half as informative but for:

- Sumeet Rastogi
- Chandeep Singh
- Albert D' Souza
- Shitij Kacker

Secretarial assistance by:

- Kanika Sharma
- Hitendra Bisht

Ever willing assistance by the publishing team M/s Jaypee Brothers Medical Publishers (P) Ltd. New Delhi, India

Contents

1

Exposures for the Complex Primary Total Hip Arthroplasty

Henry Budd, Vikas Khanduja

The purpose of this chapter is to explore the obstacles that an arthroplasty surgeon may encounter when undertaking the approach to the complex, or difficult, primary hip arthroplasty and propose a strategy to deal with the same. The complex primary hip is that where the risk of intraoperative technical difficulty, perioperative complications or risk of early failure is higher than usual and these cases invite the use of multiple techniques to achieve an adequate surgical exposure necessary to perform a successful arthroplasty. Significant bony deformation of the femur or acetabulum can occur secondary to congenital, developmental and acquired conditions resulting in axial, angular or versional abnormalities in combination with surrounding soft tissue abnormalities that require consideration when planning a surgical strategy. The principal aim of exposing the complex primary hip, like that of the routine primary hip arthroplasty, is to apply anatomical knowledge and surgical experience to safely reach the hip joint, adequately exposing the femur and acetabulum and allow controlled implantation of the prosthesis. Several key factors must be considered when deciding the most appropriate approach to use for the complex primary arthroplasty where gross anatomic distortion is often encountered, precluding the use of non-extensile approaches routinely utilized for the majority of primary hip arthroplasties. The complex hip arthroplasty often demands an extensile approach with further modifications to provide a wide exposure of the anterior and the posterior aspect of the acetabulum and the femur facilitating the performance of a femoral or pelvic osteotomy,

bone grafting and acetabular reconstruction in addition to leg lengthening. The main approaches and modifications to consider are the extended posterolateral approach, trochanteric and proximal femoral osteotomy and the triradiate exposure which can then be applied by the surgeon to individual surgical scenarios including acetabular protrusio, bone deficiency, ankylosis, limb lengthening and osteoporosis. The anterior and anterolateral approaches will not be discussed since, while they can be used for complex primary hip arthroplasty, they are not extensile and less suited to the demands of these procedures than the alternatives discussed below.

The key approaches and techniques of osteotomy will be described first followed by the specific clinical situations in which they can be applied and the techniques of exposure required for each.

APPROACHES USED FOR THE COMPLEX PRIMARY HIP ARTHROPLASTY

Posterior and Posterolateral Approaches and Modifications

This is the utility approach to the hip commonly applied to standard primary hip arthroplasty and also used for the complex primary and revision hip arthroplasty due to its extensile nature. Originally popularized by Gibson and Moore, having recognized the advantage of a potentially bloodless field, rapid exposure and limited potential muscle dennervation, the posterior approach has undergone numerous

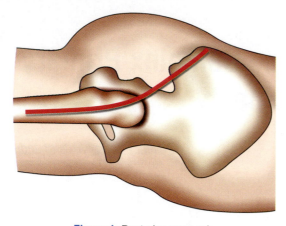

Figure 1: Posterior approach

modifications in response to the demands of both complex primary and revision arthroplasty since its original inception by Von Langenbeck in 1874 as an approach to drain suppurative arthritis.[1-3]

For the posterior approach, the patient is placed in the lateral decubitus position and secured with anterior and posterior stabilizing posts. The skin incision described by Moore in the Southern approach is placed longitudinally over the posterior third of the greater trochanter distally with the proximal limb extending in the direction of the fibers of gluteus maximus towards the posterior superior iliac spine and distally in line with the femoral shaft for 10 to 15 cm (Figure 1). After incising the skin and fat, the fascia lata is incised over the greater trochanter and split distally while proximally aponeurosis of gluteus maximus and its fibers are split and gently separated. The trochanteric bursa is encountered next, incised anteriorly and swept posteriorly with a swab to protect the sciatic nerve posteriorly exposing the short external rotators. Care is taken to protect the sciatic nerve throughout, especially important where it may be surrounded by dense fibrous scar tissue in cases where previous hip surgery has been performed or in the presence of an underlying destructive primary pathology. Dissection of the sciatic nerve is only rarely necessary given the significant added risk of iatrogenic injury. Stay sutures are placed in the piriformis tendon proximally while a retractor keeps the overhanging gluteus medius out of the operative field. The piriformis, obturator internus and gemelli

with the posterior capsule are then divided as the hip is internally rotated and the hip is dislocated in flexion, adduction and internal rotation. In certain scenarios the quadratus femoris and gluteal sling can be released from the femur to further enhance exposure through the posterior approach and to enhance achieve exposure posteriorly the gluteus maximus insertion to the femur can be incised leaving a tendinous cuff for later repair. A modification of this approach described by Shaw uses an osteotomy of the posterior third of the greater trochanter which is reflected backwards with the short external rotators, hip capsule as well as the posterior gluteus medius allowing access to the hip and reliable closure by reattaching the bony fragment.[4]

Hip dislocation can be complicated by protrusio acetabulae, the presence of abundant marginal acetabular osteophytes, significant heterotrophic ossification, Coxa Magna and surrounding soft tissue contracture. In these cases osteotomy must be performed *in situ* if dislocation cannot safely be achieved by performing an extended capsulotomy and removal of osteophytes or heterotrophic ossification. After performing the femoral osteotomy the head is removed and retractors are positioned behind the anterior and posterior wall of the acetabulum and under the transverse acetabular ligament to adequately expose the acetabulum.

Where further exposure of the anterior or posterior acetabular walls or columns is required such as with the Crowe IV high hip dislocation, the posterolateral Kocher-Langenbeck approach can be considered in preference to the routine posterior approach. This hybrid of the original approach later modified by Moore as the posterior approach and the Kocher incision is well known to pelvic and acetabular surgeons for reconstruction of acetabular fractures.[3,5] This approach is placed more anteriorly over the greater trochanter and for cases of complex primary hip arthroplasty may also require the Harris modification with a posteriorly directed third limb distally that allows posterior soft tissues to be retracted.[6]

For further exposure of the proximal femur required when there is femoral dysplasia, a narrow femoral canal or rotational deformity, a proximal femoral osteotomy is planned and the incision can be continued distally. Subsequently, one of the techniques described in the osteotomy section is utilized to expose the femur adequately.

Triradiate Exposure

This refers to a combined anterior and posterior approach using a triradiate skin and fascia incision.[23] It has been suggested for use in complex primary arthroplasty cases such as protrusio acetabuli, marked obesity, osteoporosis and ankylosis. The three equal limbs of the incision are centered over the prominence of the greater trochanter with the distal limb overlying the mid-lateral line of the femur and the two proximal limbs at 120° to this anteriorly and posteriorly (Figure 2). After completing the incision of the skin and subcutaneous fat, a 1cm wide strip of fascia lata is exposed along each limb after which it is incised. Once each fascial flap is retracted the standard anterolateral and posterior capsular exposures can be used to gain access to the hip through partial capsulotomies. Where extensive anterior and posterior capsulotomy is required for exposure meticulous repair must be performed to reduce the risk of dislocation. While devascularization of skin apices, subcutaneous tissue and fascia is a concern, in a series of 47 procedures in 46 cases, Krackow et al report satisfactory healing of the triradiate incision including a case of an auxiliary iliac crest incision for bone graft harvesting.[23] This extensive approach can be used where trochanteric osteotomy is to be

avoided, such as with morbidly obese patients, those with osteoporosis and major debilitation where the risk of reattachment failure is higher. The triradiate skin incision is, however, best avoided in patients with diabetes mellitus, fragility of the skin from steroid use or in some cases of previously scarred skin from surgery although on occasion these can be incorporated.

Direct Lateral Procedures

The continuity of the gluteus medius and the vastus lateralis over the greater trochanter has been exploited by a number of classical surgical exposures including that described by Learmonth, Hardinge as well as previously by MacFarland and Osborne who noted that the gluteus medius and vastus lateralis are in "direct functional continuity" through the thick "tendinous" periosteum covering the greater trochanter (Figure 3).[24-26] Modifications of these techniques can be similarly applied in both revision and complex primary arthroplasty surgery providing adequate exposure for both proximal femoral osteotomy and arthroplasty. The key advantage of

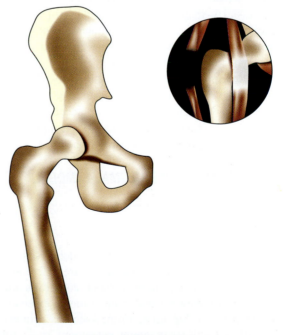

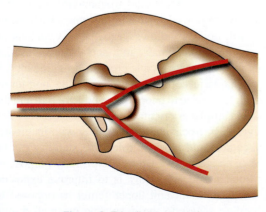

Figure 2: Triradiate approach

Figure 3: Direct lateral

these techniques is that they expose the proximal femur without the need for trochanteric osteotomy. These approaches are suitable in some complex primary hip arthroplasty situations, particularly when the surgeon is less familiar with the posterolateral approach or when they are relatively contraindicated in situations where the abductor muscles are already significantly weakened, such as in hip ankylosis.

The anterior slide can be used to expose the entire length of the femoral shaft if indicated. The continuity of the vastus lateralis and gluteus medius is maintained and proximally the common insertion is released from the anterior margin of the greater trochanter while maintaining a tendinous cuff and continued distally by subperiosteal dissection elevating the vastus lateralis from the intermuscular septum, which is maintained while perforating blood vessels, are ligated. Where a further extensile exposure of the acetabulum is required the vastus slide can be extended proximally with incorporation of the Smith-Peterson or the Henry acetabular approach.

Another useful soft tissue vastus lateralis approach described by McMinn to visualize the whole acetabulum and proximal femur utilizes an apex distal V-shaped subperiosteal flap of proximal vastus lateralis and fascia with gluteus medius and minimus reflected off the greater trochanter and proximal femur.[40] This exposes the hip capsule and following capsulotomy the entire acetabulum, without the need for a trochanteric osteotomy. An increase in leg length can also be accommodated with this approach since at closure a simple V-Y plasty of the myofascial flap is performed.

TROCHANTERIC AND PROXIMAL FEMORAL OSTEOTOMIES

Trochanteric Osteotomy

Trochanteric osteotomy has been widely used by surgeons to achieve satisfactory circumferential exposure of the hip joint without compromising soft tissue attachments and is the ultimate extensile approach to the hip joint. In the complex primary hip arthroplasty, trochanteric osteotomy is useful

not only to prepare the dysplastic femur but also to allow improved exposure of the hip capsule and the acetabulum, particularly in hips that are stiff or in cases of severe acetabular protrusio or gross proximal femoral deformity. A trochanteric osteotomy may be favored over the posterolateral approach where it is perceived that hip dislocation will be problematic with a significant risk of intraoperative femoral shaft fracture due to limited hip rotation particularly prominent in ankylosing spondylitis, acetabular protrusio and severe heterotrophic ossification where trochanteric osteotomy is followed by an *in situ* femoral neck osteotomy. However, in situations where a significant risk of heterotrophic ossification is predicted including ankylosing spondylitis, the use of preoperative radiotherapy may increase the risk of non-union of the trochanteric osteotomy and other soft tissue strategies should be considered as an alternative.

A great many modifications of the trochanteric osteotomy are described varying the extent, orientation and fixation of the osteotomy and with variable results. The basic types of trochanteric osteotomy are the simple conventional transverse transtrochanteric, the extended conventional, the Chevron (biplane), the partial trochanteric, the anterior trochanteric slide, the Stracathro and the vertical and horizontal osteotomy.[7-12] The osteotomy should provide adequate access to the proximal femur and acetabulum, allow soft tissue preservation and enable reliable stable fixation with satisfactory union rates safeguarding abductor function. The conventional trochanteric osteotomy, routinely employed by Charnley when performing hip arthroplasty allows excellent visualization of the proximal femur and acetabulum but this transtrochanteric technique presents a significant risk of trochanteric complications including non-union and migration due to unopposed abductor pull and the unstable uniplanar orientation of the osteotomy[7]. The Chevron 30° trochanteric osteotomy with its greater surface area and intrinsic rotational stability can be used as an alternative where the primary purpose of the trochanteric osteotomy is to improve exposure of the acetabulum and upper femur as opposed to improving access to the dysplastic or small femur.

The study by Weber and Stumer in 1979 compared patients with a transtrochanteric osteotomy with patients with a Chevron osteotomy and reported a 11% pseudoarthrosis rate in the conventional group and 1.5% in the Chevron group illustrating why the transtrochanteric technique is now largely historical.[13] However, there are still potential problems with the Chevron osteotomy including intraoperative fracture during fixation and the inability to place it anteriorly or posteriorly.[14]

In cases of ankylosis, a trochanteric osteotomy followed by an *in situ* neck cut exposes the proximal femur and acetabulum allowing further assessment of bone stock and deformity to be made and a better approximation of the anatomic location of the acetabulum.[15] Modification of the technique with the extended trochanteric osteotomy has lessened the risk of complications and allowed for reliable union.[9,14-20]

The trochanteric slide osteotomy described by English in 1971 solves the problem of proximal migration of the trochanter by osteotomizing the origin of the vastus lateralis muscle along with the osteotomy but this does not significantly increase access to the proximal femur and cannot be used where changes in leg length are anticipated.[21] An alternative to the trochanteric slide is the Stracathro approach, which maintains continuity of the gluteus medius and the vastus lateralis by performing a thin osteotomy of the anterior and posterior lateral greater trochanter which has the vastus lateralis and gluteus medius tendons attached proximal and distal and the short external rotators posteriorly.[11] The osteotomised fragments can then slide backwards and forwards exposing the hip, which can then be dislocated anteriorly and repair can be achieved by suturing the bony fragments with their tendinous attachments to the greater trochanter.

Proximal Femoral Osteotomy

A proximal femoral osteotomy is required where a significant proximal femoral deformity is present or femoral shortening is necessary and this can be achieved in a number of ways. The common types of proximal femoral osteotomy are the transverse osteotomy, step-cut, uniplanar or biplanar wedge and Chevron (Figures 4A and B). These may be

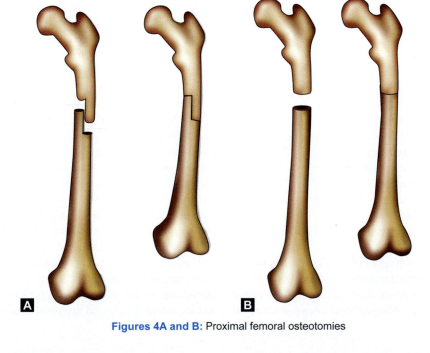

Figures 4A and B: Proximal femoral osteotomies

combined with a separate trochanteric osteotomy in some cases to assist exposure of the true acetabulum and restoration of abductor tension. Younger et al describe an extended proximal femoral osteotomy for use in revision hip surgery to remove the well-fixed femoral stem but still relevant in complex hip arthroplasty scenarios where there is significant deformity of the proximal femur.[9] This osteotomy takes the greater trochanter and proximal femur with attachment of the gluteus medius and minimus and opens on an anterolateral periosteal and muscle hinge exposing the femoral canal allowing preservation of blood supply and preventing proximal migration after reattachment.[9] Firestone describes another form of extended trochanteric osteotomy, wherein the lateral femoral cortex is osteotomized just lateral to the linea aspera and extended distally but continuity is maintained with the proximal femur.[18] In a case series of 6 patients undergoing an extended trochanteric osteotomy for complex primary hip arthroplasty Della Vale et al suggested that in selected cases, particularly where existing implants must be removed and femoral deformity must be corrected, this technique had a satisfactory rate of union and was less technically demanding than alternatives including a wedge or step-cut osteotomy.[22]

COMPLEX PRIMARY HIP CONDITIONS

Hip Dysplasia

The approach must address the following key obstacles in this condition:

- *Acetabular deficiency*
- *Femoral head subluxation or dislocation*
- *Limb length discrepancy*
- *Abnormal neurovascular structures*
- *Soft tissue contracture*
- *Excessive femoral neck-shaft anteversion*
- *Abductor dysfunction*

A patient with developmental hip dysplasia invites a multitude of important challenges to the surgeon performing a total hip arthroplasty. The hip dysplasia may be secondary to developmental dysplasia of the hip, Legg-Calve-Perthes disease and slipped upper femoral epiphysis among others. Gross anatomical distortion of the acetabulum and proximal femur can be present which must be carefully considered when planning the surgical approach that will offer maximal exposure and arthroplasty to be safely performed. The femoral head lies proximal to the true acetabulum in the high dislocation and the frequently atrophic abductor muscles therefore pass almost horizontally rather than in their normal vertical orientation.[27-29] The femoral nerve and profunda femoris artery are at significant risk of direct laceration or indirect traction injury as they pass across the patient's true acetabulum having looped backwards up to the position of the displaced femoral neck before descending[27,30] and the normal anatomical planes are absent and cautious dissection must be followed before placement of retractors around the acetabulum.[30] Rotational deformity of the proximal femur is also manifest with substantial femoral anteversion, a shortened femoral neck and posterior placement of the greater trochanter, potentially resulting in anterior dislocation if not corrected intraoperatively.[31-33] Identification of the true acetabulum is a further challenge though it is possible to identify it by opening the hip capsule and passing a finger down within the capsule through the hourglass contracture and into the true acetabulum.[30]

The Crowe classification described in 1979 is a useful guide to the technique required to achieve adequate exposure of the hip and restore the hip center while also allowing for femoral shortening and derotation.[34] This classification groups patients according to the degree of dysplasia and dislocation; and in Crowe 3 and 4, the hip joint is completely dislocated, but in the latter, also called the high dislocation, the acetabulum is insufficiently developed and more than 100% subluxation is present. Restoration of the anatomical hip center is an important goal to reduce acetabular wear rates and restore normal hip biomechanics but in the Crowe 4 completely dislocated hip this can result in significant leg lengthening and potential sciatic and femoral nerve traction injury.[35,36] The subtrochanteric and transtrochanteric approaches afford excellent exposure, allow alteration of leg length, rotational correction, restoration of the hip center and protect against nerve injury and are most suited to complex primary hip arthroplasty. The posterior approach can also be used for these cases given its extensile nature but other approaches, including the direct lateral modified Hardinge approach, have been successfully implemented for Crowe 4 dysplastic hips, however, these will frequently also require a proximal femoral osteotomy to be performed and therefore are more suited to the milder cases.[37]

The ideal subtrochanteric osteotomy will allow shortening, adjustment of the rotational alignment of the femur, access to the dysplastic proximal femur and acetabulum in addition to reliable fixation and union. Although the femur is shortened during the operation, the distalization of the femoral head to sit in the true acetabulum often results in an overall leg lengthening. The transverse subtrochanteric osteotomy described by Yasgur allows shortening and derotation to be performed and either a cemented or uncemented femoral component used.[33] Alignment and length can be determined intraoperatively by reducing the proximal femur with trial femoral component and checking bony overlap. When required, osteotomies can be re-cut which compares favorably to Chevron and step-cut osteotomies which require careful preoperative templating and planning since they are less amenable to alteration. This osteotomy can then be secured with locking plate fixation and reinforced if necessary with cables. Bruce et al have also described a subtrochanteric shortening femoral osteotomy for use with a modular femoral component, which is performed with the prosthesis *in situ* and judged by measuring the distance between the center of the femoral head and acetabular component with the leg placed under maximal tension.[38] This technique was suggested for use in patients with a relatively straight proximal femur and good bone quality where an uncemented prosthesis could be used.[38]

In some situations the dysplastic femoral canal may be too narrow at the isthmus for the smallest size femoral stem, although many manufacturers do produce specialist stems for such situations, and in these cases, adequate exposure can be achieved by splitting the femoral shaft anteriorly and posteriorly while also performing a trochanteric advancement.[39] To expose the proximal femur the vastus lateralis can

be detached proximally or the McMinn V-Y vastus lateralis procedure can be used which also enables later adjustment of abductor tension at closure.[40]

Arthroplasty for Hip Ankylosis

The approach must address the following key obstacles in this condition:
- *Identification of the true acetabulum and hip center*
- *Chronic hip abductor atrophy*
- *Defining the neck-pelvis junction*
- *Protecting the sciatic nerve and anterior neurovascular structures*
- *Leg lengthening*
- *Appropriate geometrical placement of prosthesis*

Surgical reconstruction of the spontaneously ankylosed or surgically arthrodesed hip with total joint arthroplasty requires adequate visualization of the anterior and posterior proximal femur and the site of the planned acetabulum. Challenges include not only those due to the primary disease process but also as a consequence of prior surgery.

The surgical incision will need to be planned considering the deformity present and where there is a fixed flexion deformity of 90°, the incision will curve sharply backwards at the greater trochanter in line with the deformity. While various approaches can be considered it is vital not to cause significant soft tissue damage, and abductor dennervation or devascularization through dissection in these cases since the abductors are already atrophic and a transtrochanteric approach would therefore be preferable to gain optimal acetabular exposure and also allow for leg lengthening. The transtrochanteric approach spares the remaining abductors while the posterior approach also preserves abductor function while the anterolateral and direct lateral approach risk direct abductor damage and dennervation through injury to the inferior branch of the superior gluteal nerve. Access to the femoral medullary canal is also facilitated by a trochanteric osteotomy since the greater trochanter often overlies this in these patients. Alternatively, the combined posterior and anterolateral approach has been successfully applied to gain exposure of the posterior and anterior neck respectively which can then be osteotomised from both sides in turn.[41] It may also be advisable to perform a release of the tensor fasciae lata, rectus femoris, gluteus medius and minimus through a second incision placed along the iliac crest to allow mobilization of the proximal femur and exposure of the acetabulum which can then be prepared. It must also be remembered that after prolonged flexion with fixed flexion deformity the leg must be maintained in flexion throughout the procedure to prevent femoral nerve injury.

The critical step in arthroplasty for the ankylosed hip is the osteotomy of the femoral neck that requires adequate exposure so the neck-pelvis junction can be identified and ensure that the acetabular wall is not mistaken for the edge of the femoral neck and subsequently compromised. This is achieved both by visualization and feel, where it is possible to identify the line of the femoral neck by palpating down to the lesser trochanter and pubofemoral arch prior to performing osteotomy.[42] The anterior and posterior neurovascular structures must also be protected while the osteotomy is performed 1cm from the pelvis. This is assisted by placing a large blunt retractor anterior to the neck and subperiosteal dissection posteriorly to protect the sciatic nerve.[43] After completion of the neck osteotomy attention can be turned to removal of the femoral head and subsequent acetabular preparation, both facilitated by exposure of preserved key landmarks including the acetabular fovea and obturator foramen.

Ankylosis can occur following significant heterotrophic ossification in patients with head injury where ossified material is present within soft tissue planes and can form peri-articular bony bars. The planned surgical approach must allow exposure and excision of heterotrophic ossified material and neck osteotomy and following this removal of the bony bars.

Acetabular Protrusio

The approach must address the following key obstacles in this condition:

• *Restoration of the hip center of rotation and femoral offset*

• *Risk of fracture during dislocation*
• *Leg length discrepancy*

In cases of acetabular protrusio, with medial wall deficiency and medial migration of the hip center beyond Kohler's line, the approach must allow adequate exposure of the femoral neck and performance of *in situ* osteotomy, adequate acetabular exposure and leg lengthening where superior migration of the femoral head has occurred. Such cases can be performed through posterior, posterolateral, anterolateral, direct lateral and transtrochanteric approaches successfully re-establishing the center of hip rotation and restoring leg length and offset. Exposure of the acetabulum is however best achieved with the transtrochanteric approach offering an excellent view of the anterior and posterior acetabulum, access to the femoral neck to perform osteotomy and the ability to correct abductor tension as offset and leg length is restored.

Inflammatory Arthritis

The approach must address the following key obstacles in this condition:
• *Osteoporosis and risk of intraoperative fracture*
• *Acetabular and femoral component orientation*
• *Difficult dislocation*
• *Postoperative heterotrophic ossification*

Many conditions are responsible for inflammatory arthritis affecting, among other joints, the hip, resulting in degenerative change. These include rheumatoid arthritis, ankylosing spondylitis, systemic lupus erythematosus, chondrocalcinosis and gout amongst many others.

In juvenile rheumatoid arthritis, care must be taken to avoid femoral fracture during hip dislocation due to coexisting osteoporosis, and an adequate capsulotomy or in some cases total capsulectomy and possibly *in situ* femoral neck osteotomy is necessary to dislocate the femoral head without applying a significant rotational force. Extensive soft tissue contracture release will also assist safe dislocation of the femoral head. The presence of osteoporosis can also lead to fragmentation of the greater trochanter during surgery if a transtrochanteric approach is utilized as is often necessary in cases where the proximal femoral canal is difficult to enter, but where possible the posterior, direct lateral or anterolateral approach are more suitable for these patients.

In patients with ankylosing spondylitis attention to accurate patient positioning in the lateral decubitus position with appreciation of the presence or absence of the normal lumbar lordosis is crucial to achieving appropriate acetabular orientation as well as a wide exposure. Hip dislocation can be difficult in some cases and may necessitate a planned *in situ* neck osteotomy after dislocation is attempted following iliopsoas tenotomy, partial or complete capsulectomy and release of soft tissue adhesions. A trochanteric osteotomy can be useful to achieve adequate circumferential acetabular visualization since it may not be possible to reliably expose the femoral neck using either the anterolateral or posterior approach which can subsequently lead to a difficult *in situ* osteotomy in severe cases and potentially removal of some acetabular wall to identify and cut the neck. This however must be balanced against the risk of postoperative non-union of the greater trochanter if postoperative irradiation is planned to reduce the risk of heterotrophic ossification in these cases. Fluoroscopy can also be used to assist identification of the femoral neck and to perform the osteotomy, although this should not be necessary with a carefully planned surgical approach such as the transtrochanteric, posterolateral or even combined posterior and anterolateral.

Conversion Primary Hip Arthroplasty for Proximal Femoral Fracture

The approach must address the following key obstacles in this condition:

Removal of Metalwork

Adequate access to the proximal femur for broaching/burring: Failure of metalwork following a proximal femoral fracture ultimately results in a complex primary total hip arthroplasty. The chosen approach must be extensile distally and allow removal of metalwork from the lateral femur achieved by subperiosteal dissection and elevation of vastus lateralis, access to the often medialized proximal femur for broaching and removal of dense sclerotic bone within the canal and reattachment of the malunited greater trochanter and attached abductors.

REFERENCES

1. Gibson A. Posterior exposure of the hip joint. JBJS 1950;32B:183-6.
2. Moore A. The Moore self-locking Vitallium prosthesis in fresh femoral neck fractures. A new low posterior approach (the southern exposure). American Academy of Orthopaedic Surgeons Instructional Course Lectures 1957;16:309-21.
3. Langenbeck, Von B. Ueber die Schusverletzungen des Huftgelenks. Archiv fur Klinische Chirurgie 1874;16:263.
4. Shaw J. Experience with a modified posterior approach to the hip joint. J Arthroplasty 1991;6:11.
5. Mehlman C, Miess L, Dipasquale T. Hypenated history: the Kocher-Langbeck surgical approach. Journal of Orthopaedic Trauma 2000;14(1):60-4.
6. Harris W. Advances in surgical technique for total hip replacement. CORR 1980;146:188.
7. Charnley J, Ferreira A. Transplantation of the greater trochanter in arthoplasty of the hip. JBJS 1964;46B(2):191.
8. Engh C Jr, McAuley J, McAuley Sr. Surgical approaches for revision total hip replacement surgery: the anterior trochanteric slide and the extended conventional osteotomy. Instructional Course Lectures 1999;48:3-8.
9. Younger T, Bradford M, Magnus R, et al. Extended proximal femoral osteotomy. J Arthroplasty 1995; 10:329-38.
10. Wroblewski B, Shelley P. Reattachment of the greater trochanter after hip replacement. JBJS 1985(67B):736.
11. McLauchlan J. The Stracathro approach to the hip. JBJS(Br) 1984;66(B):30-1.
12. Dall D. Exposure of the hip by anterior osteotomy of the greater trochanter. JBJS 1986;30B:382-6.
13. Weber B, Stuhmer G. Improvements in total hip prosthesis implantation technique: a cement proof seal for the lower medullary canal and a dihedral self-stabilising trochanteric osteotomy. Arch Orthop Trauma Surg 1979;93:185-9.

14. Callaghan JJ. Difficult primary total hip arthroplasty: selected surgical approaches. Instr Course Lect 2000; 49:13-21.

15. Blackley HR, Rorabeck CH. Extensile exposures for revision hip arthroplasty. Clin Orthop 2000;381: 77-87.

16. Berry D, Muller M. Chevron osteotomy and single wire reattachment of the greater trochanter in primary and revision hip total hip arthroplasty. Clin Orthop 1993;294:155-61.

17. Chen W, McAuley J, Engh C, et al. Extended slide trochanteric slide osteotomy for revision total hip arthroplasty. JBJS (Am) 2000;82:1215-9.

18. Firestone T, Hedley A. Extended proximal femoral osteotomy for severe acetabular protrusion following total hip arthroplasty: a technical note. J Arthroplasty 1997;12:344-5.

19. Head W, Mallory T, Berklacich F, et al. Extensile exposure of the hip for revision arthroplasty. J Arthroplasty 1987;2:265-73.

20. Masterson EL, Masri BA, Duncan CP. Surgical approaches in revision hip replacement. J Am Acad Orthop Surg 1998;6:84-92.

21. TA English, The trochanteric approach to the hip for prosthetic replacement, J Bone Joint Surg 57A 1975. p. 1128.

22. Della Vale C, et al. Extended Trochanteric Osteotomy in Complex Primary Total Hip Arthroplasty. A Brief Note. J Bone Joint Surg Am 2003;85:2385-90.

23. Krackow K, Steinman H, Cohn B, et al. Clinical experience with a triradiate exposure of the hip for difficult total hip arthroplasty. J Arthroplasty 1988;3: 267.

24. Learmonth ID, Allen PE. The omega lateral approach to the hip. JBJS 1996;78B:559-61.

25. Hardinge K. The direct lateral approach to the hip. JBJS 1982;64B:17-9.

26. Mcfarland B, Osborne G. Approach to the hip. A suggested improvement of the Kocher's method. JBJS 1954;36B:364.

27. Callaghan J, Rosenberg A, Rubash H. The Adult Hip. Lippincott Williams and Wilkins.

28. Haddad F, et al. Primary Total Replacement of the Dysplastic Hip. AAOS Instructional Course Lectures 2000;29:23-36.

29. McCarthy J, Bono J, Lee J. The Difficult Femur. AAOS Instructional Course Lectures 2000;49:63-9.

30. Blackley HR, Rorabeck CH. Extensile exposures for revision hip arthroplasty. Clin Orthop 2000;381: 77-87.

31. Charnley J, Feagin JA. Low-friction arthroplasty in congenital subluxation of the hip. Clin Orthop 1973; 91:98.

32. Harris WH. Total hip replacement for congenital dysplasia of the hip: technique. In Harris WH(ed): The Hip: Proceedings of the Second Open Scientific Meeting of The Hip Society. CV Mosby, St Louis, p 251.

33. Yasgur DJ, Stutchin SA, Adler EM, DiCesare PE. Subtrochanteric femoral shortening osteotomy in total hip arthroplasty for high riding developmental dislocation of the hip. J Arthroplasty 1997;12:880-8.

34. Crowe J, Mani V, Ranawat C. Total hip replacement in congenital dislocation and dysplasia of the hip. JBJS 1979;61A:15-23.

35. Bernasek T, et al. Total hip arthroplasty requiring subtrochanteric osteotomy for developmental hip dysplasia. The Journal of Arthroplasty 2007;22(6): 145-50.

36. Pagnano M, et al. The effect of superior placement of the acetabular component on the rate of loosening after total hip arthroplasty. Long-term results in patients who have crowe Type-II congenital dysplasia of the hip. JBJS 1996;78:1004-14.

37. Makita H. Results on total hip arthroplasties with femoral shortening for Crowe's group IV dislocated hips. The Journal of Arthroplasty 2007; 22(1):32-8.

38. Bruce W, et al. A new technique of subtrochanteric shortening in total hip arthroplasty. The Journal of Arthroplasty 2000;15(5):617-26.

39. Eskelinen A, et al. Cementless total hip arthroplasty in patients with high congenital hip dislocation. JBJS (Am) 2006;88:80-91.

40. McMinn D, Roberts P, Forward G. A new approach to the hip for revision surgery. JBJS 1991;73B:899-901.

41. Idulhaq M, et al. Total hip arthroplasty for treatment of fused hip with 90 degree flexion deformity. The Journal of Arthroplasty 2010;25(3):498.

42. Bhan S, Eachempati K, Malhotra R. Primary cementless total hip arthroplasty for bony ankylosis in patients with ankylosing spondylitis. The Journal of Arthroplasty 2008;23(6):859-66.

43. Morsi E. Total Hip Arthroplasty for fused hips; planning and techniques. The Journal of Arthroplasty 2007;22(6):871-5.

2 | Total Hip Replacement in Avascular Necrosis Hip

Rajesh Bawari, Shivan Marya

Avascular necrosis (AVN) of the femoral head is a common musculoskeletal disorder. Although patients are initially asymptomatic, AVN of the femoral head usually progresses to joint destruction which may eventually require total hip replacement (THR). This requirement may arise earlier than later, usually before the fifth decade.Femoral head has precarious blood supply making it prone to infarction and AVN. Blood supply enters through very narrow spaces, which when compromised by trauma or a disease process leads to ischemic necrosis. The collateral circulation is inadequate to take over tissue perfusion. AVN of femoral head usually involves a part and rarely the entire head. Histologically this entails disappearance of osteocytes from their lacunae with subsequent attempt at revascularization that extends inward from the adjacent viable bone which is very slow. Hyperemia of surrounding viable bone causes local osteoporosis, while infarcted bone retains its density and thus appears whiter or denser on radiographs. As vessels approach necrotic area, osteoclastic resorption of bone at the interface may weaken the femoral head so much that a portion of it will collapse, resulting in alteration in the spherical shape of femoral head. An irregular articular surface now present sets the stage for painful degenerative arthritis.

AVN of femoral head may be idiopathic. The known common causes of AVN are:
- Trauma
  - Fracture neck of femur
  - Dislocation hip
- Large doses of steroids
- Gout
- Alcoholism
- Diabetes
- Sickle cell anemia
- Decompression sickness
- Gaucher's disease
- Perthes' disease
- Following transplant surgeries (3% in patients of cardiac transplant surgery and up to 25% of patients following renal transplant).
- In pregnancy
- Systemic lupus erythematosus,
- Chemoradiotherapy exposure,
- Myeloproliferative disorders, and
- Thalassemias.[1-5]

STAGING OF AVN FEMORAL HEAD

AVN of the femoral head is commonly staged by the University of Pennsylvania System,[6] proposed by Steinberg.

Stage 0: Normal MRI
Stage I: Abnormal MRI, Normal Radiograph

A. Mild (<15% of head involvement)
B. Moderate (15 to 30% head involvement)
C. Severe (>30% head involvement)

Stage II: Abnormal Radiograph Showing Cystic and Sclerotic Changes in the Femoral Head

A. Mild (<15% of head involvement)
B. Moderate (15 to 30% head involvement)
C. Severe (>30% head involvement)

Stage III: Subchondral Collapse Producing a Crescent Sign

A. Mild (<15% of articular surface involvement)
B. Moderate (15 to 30% articular surface involvement)
C. Severe (>30% articular involvement)

Stage IV: Flattening of the Femoral Head

A. Mild (<15% of articular surface and <2 mm depression)
B. Moderate (15 to 30% of articular surface or 2 to 4 mm depression)
C. Severe (>30% articular surface or > 4 mm depression)

Stage V: Joint Narrowing with or Without Acetabular Involvement

A. Mild
B. Moderate
C. Severe

Stage VI: Advanced Degenerative Changes

Approximately 30% of the silent hips will go on to collapse, in contrast symptomatic hip almost uniformly progresses to further collapse without treatment. The collapse rates approach greater than 85%, even if first seen in the earliest stages. Treatment plan for the asymptomatic AVN is controversial. Better outcomes have been demonstrated with core decompression for very early stages of AVN.

TREATMENT OF AVN FEMORAL HEAD

Treatment of AVN of femoral head may be non-operative or operative depending on the stage at which it is detected. Non-operative treatments include rest, non-weight-bearing exercises, protected weight-bearing, medications etc. Operative treatments include core decompression with or without bone grafting, hemi-resurfacing, fusion, osteotomy, hemi-arthroplasty, as well as total hip arthroplasty (THA).

Treatment: University of Pennsylvania Stages I, II, and III

The primary goal in managing early avascular necrosis (AVN) of the hip is pain control and prevention of femoral head collapse. This is accomplished with early diagnosis and early initiation of treatment. Since there is no universally successful prophylactic intervention for AVN of femoral head, many continue to go on to femoral head collapse and require hip arthroplasty. Medications like anticoagulants and bisphosphonates have been tried with variable results.

Surgical treatment for early stages of AVN of femoral head includes core decompression with or without bone grafting (Figures 1 and 2). Core decompression of the hip is usually employed before collapse of the femoral head and/or neck to delay or avoid joint replacement surgery. It is aimed at preserving the structure of the femoral head besides relieving pain associated with AVN of femoral head. There is adequate evidence that core decompression is effective in treating early stages (I or II) of AVN of the hip. Simank et al have compared intertrochanteric osteotomy to core decompression.[7] They revealed survival rates of 74% after the osteotomy and 78% after core decompression 6 years postoperatively in early, pre-collapse stages (p = 0.819).

von Stechow and Drees (2007) have recommended core decompression as the treatment of choice for early small and medium-sized pre-collapse lesions of AVN of femoral head.[8] Osteotomies and bone grafting procedures were to be utilized in medium pre-collapse, as well as in small post-collapse lesions. Cartilage lesions of the femoral head allowed limited femoral resurfacing arthroplasty. In patients where the acetabulum revealed cartilage lesions, total hip replacement was suggested.

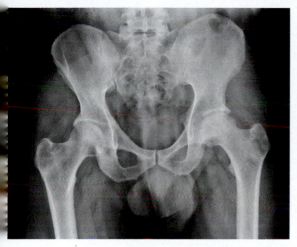

Figure 1: AVN left hip with core decompression

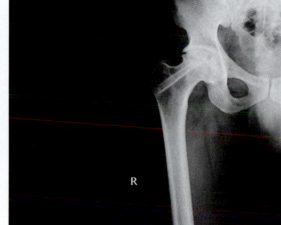

Figure 2: AVN right hip with failed fibular grafting

The effectiveness of core decompression has been peer-reviewed in more than 40 studies. In general, this treatment is most successful for patients with early stage, small- and medium-sized lesions, before collapse of the femoral head. Various methods of non-vascularized bone grafting have been used. Results have varied with these procedures; however, a 60 to 80% success rate has been achieved at 5 to 10-year follow-up.

The use of a free vascularized fibular graft in the treatment of osteonecrosis has been popularized by some as an excellent option to delay the need for total joint arthroplasty.[9-12] However, the procedure has limitations. The grafting procedure is lengthy, requiring microvascular skills on the part of the surgeon and a potentially longer hospital stay. Complications can occur at the donor site besides the grafted site and can cause appreciable patient morbidity. Forty-three percent of patients have weakness in the great toe, 11% have ankle pain, and 5% have a major complication.[13] It also has potential for failure and a need for conversion to hip arthroplasty.

The rate at which free vascularized fibular grafts must be converted to total hip replacement ranges from 8% at a mean duration of follow-up of 4.7 years[14] to 27% at a mean of 4.2 years.[15] Given the relatively reduced functional outcome after conversion of a failed free vascularized fibular graft to total joint

arthroplasty and the complications associated with the operation, the overall improvement in outcome following this technique may not be as attractive as initially portrayed with the data on graft survivorship alone.

Treatment: University of Pennsylvania Stages III, IV and V

Resurfacing arthroplasty has been tried as a bone conserving surgery for later stages of disease. This may be limited resurfacing/hemisurface replacement and femoral and acetabular resurfacing arthroplasty. This is an alternative to total hip replacement in certain subgroup of patients (e.g. sickle cell anemia, post-transplantation, chronic alcoholism) that have not fared as well with total hip replacement. Hemi-surface replacement has been used as an interim solution in Types III and IV (University of Penn-sylvania AVN staging). Mont et al have restricted its use to patients with relatively healthy acetabular cartilage.[16] Though most patients pursue high activity sports groin pain has been reported in about 20% of the patients.

Femoral and acetabular hip resurfacing was proposed to be a more permanent procedure. One essential prerequisite being adequate femoral head bone stock to carry out surface replacement. This can be checked both on preoperative radiographs and at the time of surgery. Surface replacement results are poor in patients who are tall, of female gender and who have femoral cysts greater than 1 cm. Patients who have been receiving corticosteroids have very soft bone. These patients are poor candidates for acetabular cup fixation in surface replacement, which usually does not have option to augment cup anchorage.

Some of the metal on metal surface replacement implants have fallen into disrepute and have been withdrawn from the market because of high metal ion concentration in blood. The Birmingham Hip Resurfacing (BHR) system (Smith & Nephew Inc., Memphis, TN, USA), the Cormet 2000 Hip Resurfacing System (Corin USA, Tampa, FL, USA) and the Wright Medical Technologies (Arlington, TX, USA), Conserve Plus Hip System are approved for use by USFDA where in indicated.

In surface replacement a mismatch between the size of the femoral prosthesis and the acetabulum may contribute to unfavorable results. That is why it is important that sizes be available in at least 2 mm increments for proper fixation and favorable tribology. Concerns over metal ions released following surface replacement have restricted the choice of this articulation to young male patients.

Smith and colleagues (2010) compared the clinical and radiological outcomes and complication rates of surface replacement hip and total hip arthroplasty (THA).[17] A systematic review was undertaken of all published (Medline, CINAHL, AMED, EMBASE) and unpublished or gray literature research databases up to January 2010. Clinical and radiological outcomes as well as complications of surface replacement hip were compared to those of THA using various statistical parameters. The meta-analysis revealed better or equal functional outcomes following surface replacement hip compared to following THA. However there were statistically significantly greater incidence of heterotopic ossification, aseptic loosening, and revision surgery with surface replacement hip. The authors concluded that, surface replacement hip may have better functional outcomes than THA, but the increased risks of heterotopic ossification, aseptic loosening, and revision surgery following surface replacement

hip indicate that THA is superior in terms of implant survival.

Garbuz and associates (2010) conducted a prospective randomized clinical trial to compare clinical outcomes of resurfacing versus large-head metal-on-metal THA.[18] These researchers randomized 107 patients deemed eligible for resurfacing arthroplasty to have either resurfacing or standard THA. Patients were assessed for quality-of-life outcomes using various functional scores. The minimum follow-up was 0.8 years (mean of 1.1 years; range of 0.8 to 2.2 years). Of the 73 patients followed at least 1 year, both groups reported improvement in quality of life on all outcome measures. There was no difference in quality of life between the 2 arms in the study. Serum levels of cobalt and chromium were measured in a subset of 30 patients. In both groups cobalt and chromium was elevated compared to baseline. Patients receiving a large-head metal-on-metal total hip had elevated ion levels compared to the resurfacing arm of the study. At 1 year, the median serum cobalt increased 46-fold from baseline in patients in the large-head total hip group, while the median serum chromium increased 10-fold. At 1 year, serum cobalt was 10-fold higher and serum chromium 2.6-fold higher than in the resurfacing arm. Due to these excessively high metal ion levels, the authors recommended against further use of this particular large-head total hip replacement.

Two papers reported on the Cormet 2000 hip resurfacing system in the same patient population.[19,20] The earlier report concludes that the resurfacing patients had equal overall clinical success with the ceramic-on-ceramic THA patients in terms of a composite score including Harris Hip Score, 'radiographic evidence of success', absence of device related complications and absence of revision; however, the MoM hip resurfacing group had substantially more revisions (7.1% vs 1.9%) in a shorter follow-up time frame.[12] Revisions were primarily due to femoral neck fractures and femoral component loosening. The THA group was the historical control. The latter report assessed the Harris Hip Score at specific time-points over two-year follow-up in the same two groups of patients, concluding that while there were differences early on, with the THA group doing better at six weeks and the MoM hip resurfacing group doing better at six months, there was no difference at 12 or 24 months with > 90% of both groups scoring in the excellent range.[19,20]

There has been increasing concern in the literature about blood metal ion levels as a result of wear from metal on metal hip replacements, in both hip resurfacing and THA. While there is no safe or toxic level of chromium and cobalt in the blood, the concern about increased levels ranges from local tissue toxicity, to chromosomal damage and malignant cellular transformation.[21-24] The four publications that focused on this topic all studied patients with BHR. One study found that both hip resurfacing and metal-on-metal THA patients with small diameter (28 mm) heads had similar chromium and cobalt levels, both higher than healthy controls without metal implants.[25] Another study compared unilateral MoM BHR, bilateral MoM BHR with metal-on-polyethylene THA and ceramic-on-ceramic THA.[26] They report the highest chromium and cobalt ion levels with both types of MoM hip replacement, smaller elevation for the metal-on-polyethylene group, and negligible levels for the ceramic-on-ceramic group. A third study again reported increased ion levels for patients with MoM hip resurfacing implants; however, they found that as the femoral component size increased, ion levels decreased, implying that with less friction and wear there is less release of ions.[27] The fourth study found enhanced lymphocyte activity for nickel, but not for chromium and cobalt; there was no difference for patients with and without pseudotumors (a cystic or solid mass relating to resurfaced hip), although the pseudotumor group was very small (n=10).[28]

TOTAL HIP ARTHROPLASTY

Total hip arthroplasty is indicated for patients with advanced AVN (University of Pennsylvania Stages IVA–VIC) unresponsive to conservative management. In these more advanced stages, joint preserving procedures are associated with less predictable results. Relative contraindications for total hip arthroplasty in AVN hip include patients in whom there is a high likelihood of the condition

responding to either conservative management or low morbidity joint preserving procedures such as core decompression, particularly in young patients.

The perception that the results of total hip replacement in patients with osteonecrosis are inferior to the results of total hip replacement in patients with osteoarthritis is not true anymore. This thought process is based on older literature, or long-term studies evaluating older implants and bearing surfaces.[29-36] Surgeons hence may not delay total hip replacement unnecessarily, or consider joint preserving procedures at a stage where these interventions may not be effective. Cementless techniques have become popular (Figure 3). The advantages are reduced bone removal, shorter operation time, and possibly the potential of easier revision.

More recent studies with better implants, bearing surfaces, and surgical techniques have demonstrated total hip replacement results much closer to those of patients with osteoarthritis,[37-41] and superior to results of joint preserving procedures and other forms of arthroplasty in these patients. Lins et al[42] reported 81% of femoral components and 97% of acetabular components were stable at mean follow-up of 60 months following uncemented fixation, while Mont et al[38] reported good to excellent results in 94% of patients at short-term follow-up.

Kim et al analyzed the survival of hybrid and cementless metal on poly THRs in young patients less than 50 years of age.[43] These were followed up for an average of 18 years. In their series, patients with osteonecrosis of the femoral head, the overall survival of the femoral stem was 96% at 20 years. The majority of patients in the series continued to participate in high-demand activities. The etiology and the level of activity did not seem to affect the longevity of fixation of acetabular and femoral components. Wear and bearing failure remained a significant concern, and newer alternative bearings were suggested for an increased lifespan from the entire prosthetic unit. According to Kim et al, recent literature suggested higher survival rates of cementless femoral stems to cemented implants in younger patients. The average rate of failure for cemented femoral components was 3.5 times higher than for porous-coated femoral components.

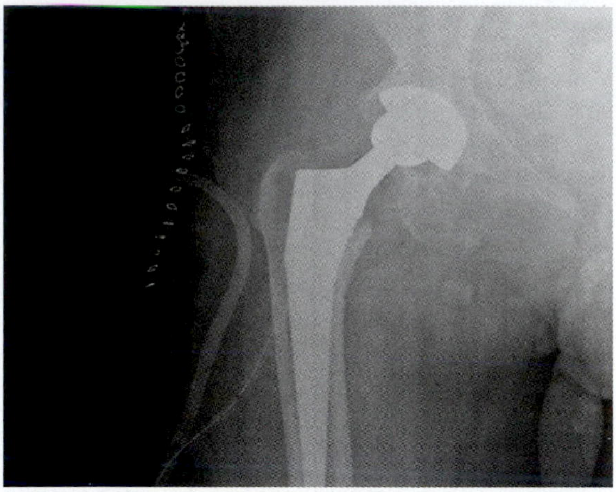

Figure 3: Postoperative pictures of AVN with degenerative arthritis right hip replaced by uncemented metal on polyethylene articulation

In recent years, there had been renewed interest in metal-on-metal bearing surfaces for total joint arthroplasty. This was for younger and more active patients who face the possibility of multiple revision procedures during their lifetime. In the long-term, the second-generation all-metal prostheses have demonstrated lower friction and wear rates than metal-on-polyethylene bearing surfaces. Recent studies reported that the second-generation metal-on-metal hip replacement prostheses exhibit a lower rate of acetabular revision and loosening than what was with previous metal-on-metal designs and that they had no more acetabular loosening or osteolysis than what was with metal-on-polyethylene articulations for follow-up periods of 5 to 10 years (Figures 4A and B). However, concern regarding metal ion release has led to withdrawal of many of these designs.

Another alternative to standard polyethylene is alumina-on-alumina ceramic. When comparing hard-on-hard bearings, the ceramic-on-ceramic coupling has several theoretical advantages over metal-on-metal. Because of the ceramic's extremely low coefficient of friction and its potential for superior wear resistance, these couples promise wear rates that are appreciably less than polyethylene-on-metal and metal-on-metal couples.

Available literature indicates that alumina-on-alumina ceramic couplings are a viable alternative to metal-on-polyethylene designs (Figures 5A and B). The combination of new high quality ceramic acetabular and femoral bearing is with hip systems that have achieved long-term stable fixation can result in a substantial increase in the longevity of fixation for implants especially in the younger and more active patients.

Millar et al demonstrated significant clinical improvements at a mean follow-up of 34 months with no significant difference between osteonecrosis and osteoarthritis groups at similar follow-up using ceramic-on-ceramic articulation.[44] The use of ceramic-on-ceramic interfaces in young, active patients may decrease wear and lower the rate of aseptic loosening of the implant and appears to be an attractive alternative to the use of conventional cobalt chromium on polyethylene or metal on metal bearings. Issues surrounding ceramic bearings include fracture, microseparation, impingement, and fewer intraoperative modular component designs were not encountered by them. This was probably because of dramatic improvements made in the third-generation manufacturing process and the design of ceramic components.

A technology assessment of hip implants by the Institute for Clinical effectiveness and health policy (Augustovsky et al, 2006) found that the clinical trials comparing ceramic against conventional prostheses found no significant differences in the revision rate among the different types of prostheses.[45] In case series of patients with the ceramic prosthesis, reported revision rates at 10 years were less than 10%, which is considered within acceptable limits and comparable to those reported for conventional prostheses. Similar results have been reported for metal on metal hip prostheses, where randomised controlled trials with follow-up up to 5 years found no differences between metal on metal and conventional prostheses in effectiveness and complication rates (Augustovsky et al, 2006). The assessment noted that, although there are some reports of an increase in cancer in persons with metal on metal hip prostheses, there are other reports

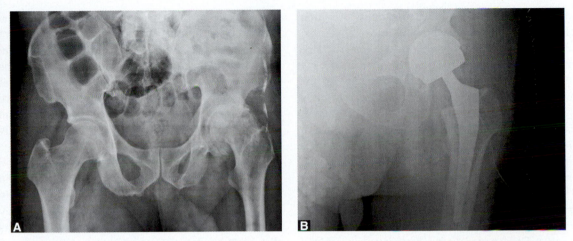

Figures 4A and B: Preoperative and postoperative pictures of AVN with degenerative arthritis left hip replaced by uncemented metal on metal articulation

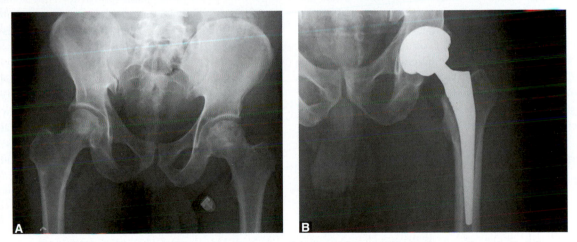

Figures 5A and B: Preoperative and postoperative pictures of bilateral AVN with degenerative arthritis left hip replaced by uncemented ceramic-on-ceramic articulation

evaluating metal on metal prostheses with follow-up up to 28 years that have found no increase in the incidence of any cancer.

The Pinnacle Complete Acetabular Hip System (DePuy Orthopaedics Inc) is the first to combine a ceramic ball and a metal socket.

There has been much debate in the literature regarding the long-term survival of a total hip prosthesis in patients with osteonecrosis. The revision rate has been reported to range from 0% at 5.8 years of follow-up[46] to 37% at eight years of follow-up.[47] Much of the poor survivorship of hips in this group of patients has been blamed on the young age of the patients rather than on the pathologic process of osteonecrosis.[48] However, the different causes of osteonecrosis have been shown to affect functional outcome after total hip arthroplasty, with corticosteroid and alcohol-induced osteonecrosis associated with the worst outcome.[46,49]

Osteonecrosis patients who suffer from sickle cell anemia have been noted to have very high rates of both infection and aseptic loosening compared with total hip arthroplasty for other conditions.[50] Additionally, sickle cell anemia creates perioperative challenges that may lead to higher rates of perioperative morbidity and mortality. Perioperative blood loss may worsen these patients' underlying anemia and lead to sickle cell crisis, including acute lung syndrome, bone crisis, and gastrointestinal complications. Development of acute lung syndrome in these patients presents treatment dilemmas due to the difficult differential diagnosis like pulmonary involvement by fat or pulmonary embolism.

There is limited literature evaluating the outcomes and complications of patients undergoing total hip arthroplasty for osteonecrosis secondary to Gaucher's disease. These patients often have extensive osteonecrosis throughout not only the femoral head, but also the entire proximal femur, and often the acetabulum as well. In reviewing the limited studies evaluating outcomes for this subgroup of patients with osteonecrosis, there does appear to be a higher rate of loosening in these individuals. The important elements of preoperative planning are the evaluation of medical comorbidities; the determination of surgical risks and preoperative medical or speciality consultation as indicated.

THR in Patients Following Vascularized Fibular Graft

A study by Davis et al raises concern that the outcome of total hip arthroplasty in patients who previously underwent a free vascularized fibular graft for the treatment of osteonecrosis of the femoral head may be worse than that in patients without previous free vascularized fibular grafting.[51] They recommended intraoperative use of a high-speed burr to improve the alignment of the femoral component by removing more of the residual graft. However, this technique does increase intraoperative blood loss and operative time. They analyzed three different types of stems, viz. a straight stem, a tapered stem without the use of a high-speed burr to remove residual graft and a tapered stem with the use of a high-speed burr to remove residual graft. The worst alignment (mean, 6.7° of varus)

was seen in the tapered-stem group when a burr was not used; an intermediate quality of alignment was seen with insertion of a straight stem without removal of residual graft (mean, 3.5° of varus). The best alignment was seen when a tapered stem was inserted after a high-speed burr was used to remove residual graft (mean, 0.4° of valgus). The mean postoperative scores at three years were significantly worse in patients who had undergone a previous free vascularized fibular graft (p = 0.03).

Similar suspicion was expressed by Berend et al in their study of patients who had total hip arthroplasty following free vascularized fibular grafting.[52] They demonstrated in their cohort of sixty-nine patients that the Harris hip score only improved from a mean of 63 prior to total hip arthroplasty to a mean of 77.4 at the time of the most recent follow-up. They noted that 38% of their patients achieved a poor result following total hip replacement after failure of a free vascularized fibular graft.

The present consensus regarding THR in AVN femoral head is use of uncemented implants. Metal on polyethylene articulations are still commonly used, however, ceramic on polyethylene/ceramic on ceramic are gaining favor. Metal on metal articulations have again fallen into disfavor because of unacceptably high metal ion levels in the blood with some popular designs.

REFERENCES

1. Mont MA, Hungerford DS. Non-traumatic avascular necrosis of the femoral head. J Bone Joint Surg Am 1995;77(3):459-74.
2. Aaron RK. Osteonecrosis: etiology, pathophysiology, and diagnosis. In: Callahan JJ, Rosenberg AG, Rubash HE, (Eds): The Adult Hip. Philadelphia, PA: Lippincott-Raven Publishers; 1998:451-6.
3. Milner PF, Kraus AP, Sebes JI, et al. Sickle cell disease as a cause of osteonecrosis of the femoral head. N Engl J Med 1991;325(21):1476-81.
4. Barden RM. Osteonecrosis of the femoral head. Orthop Nurs 1985;4(4):45-51.
5. Patial RK, Bansal SK, Kashyap S, Negi A. Drug interaction-induced osteonecrosis of femoral head. J Assoc Physicians India 1990;38(6):446-7.

6. Stemberg ME, Hoyken GD, Steinberg DR. A quantative system for staging Aroscular Necrosis, J Bone Joint Surg. Br. 1995;77(1):34-41.

7. Simank HG, Brocai DR, Brill C, Lukoschek M Comparison of results of core decompression and intertrochanteric osteotomy for nontraumatic osteonecrosis of the femoral head using Cox regression and survivorship analys. J Arthroplasty 2001;16(6):790.

8. von Stechow D, Drees P. Surgical treatment concepts for femoral head necrosis. Orthopade 2007;36(5):451-7.

9. Urbaniak JR, Coogan PG, Gunneson EB, Nunley JA. Treatment of osteonecrosis of the femoral head with free vascularized fibular grafting. A long-term follow-up study of one hundred and three hips. J Bone Joint Surg Am 1995;77:681-94.

10. Malizos KN, Soucacos PN, Beris AE. Osteonecrosis of the femoral head. Hip salvaging with implantation of a vascularized fibular graft. Clin Orthop Relat Res 1995;314:67-75.

11. Sotereanos DG, Plakseychuk AY, Rubash HE. Free vascularized fibula grafting for the treatment of osteonecrosis of the femoral head. Clin Orthop Relat Res 1997;344:243-56.

12. Yoo MC, Chung DW, Hahn CS. Free vascularized fibula grafting for the treatment of osteonecrosis of the femoral head. Clin Orthop Relat Res 1992;277:128-38.

13. Tang CL, Mahoney JL, McKee MD, Richards RR, Waddell JP, Louie B. Donor site morbidity following vascularized fibular grafting. Microsurgery 1998;18:383-86.

14. Soucacos PN, Beris AE, Malizos K, Koropilias A, Zalavras H, Dailiana Z. Treatment of avascular necrosis of the femoral head with vascularized fibular transplant. Clin Orthop Relat Res 2001;386:120-30.

15. Louie BE, McKee MD, Richards RR, Mahoney JL, Waddell JP, et al. Treatment of osteonecrosis of the femoral head by free vascularized fibular grafting: an analysis of surgical outcome and patient health status. Can J Surg 1999;42:274-83.

16. Mont, Michael A; Delanois, Ronald E; Quesada, Mario J; Childress, Lorenzo. Techniques in Orthopaedics: Femoral and Acetabular Surface Replacement and Hemi-Surface Replacement for Osteonecrosis of the Hip 2008;23(1):65-73.

17. Smith TO, Nichols R, Donell ST, Hing CB. The clinical and radiological outcomes of hip resurfacing versus total hip arthroplasty: a meta-analysis and systematic review. Acta Orthop 2010;81(6):684-95.

18. Garbuz DS, Tanzer M, Greidanus NV, et al. The John Charnley Award: metal-on-metal hip resurfacing versus large-diameter head metal-on-metal total hip arthroplasty: a randomized clinical trial. Clin Orthop ERelat Res 2010;468(2):318-25.

19. Stulberg BN, Fitts SM, Bowen AR, Zadzilka JD. Early return to function after hip resurfacing is it better than contemporary total hip arthroplasty? J Arthroplasty 2009.

20. Stulberg BN, Trier KK, Naughton M, Zadzilka JD. Results and lessons learned from a United States hip resurfacing investigational device exemption trial. J Bone Joint Surg Am 2008;(90)3:21-6.

21. Parry MC, Bhabra G, Sood A, et al. Thresholds for indirect DNA damage across cellular barriers for orthopaedic biomaterials. Biomaterials 31(16):4477-83.

22. Keegan GM, Learmonth ID, Case CP. A systematic comparison of the actual, potential, and theoretical health effects of cobalt and chromium exposures from industry and surgical implants. Crit Rev Toxicol 2008;38(8):645-74.

23. Cobb AG, Schmalzreid TP. The clinical significance of metal ion release from cobalt-chromium metal-on-metal hip joint arthroplasty. Proc Inst Mech Eng H 2006;220(2):385-98.

24. Nyren O, McLaughlin JK, Gridley G, et al. Cancer risk after hip replacement with metal implants: a population-based cohort study in Sweden. J Natl Cancer Inst 1995;87(1):28-33.

25. Moroni A, Savarino L, Cadossi M, Baldini N, Giannini S. Does ion release differ between hip resurfacing and metal-on-metal THA? Clin Orthop Relat Res 2008;466(3):700-707.

26. Hart AJ, Skinner JA, Winship P, et al. Circulating levels of cobalt and chromium from metal-on-metal hip replacement are associated with CD8+ T-cell lymphopenia. J Bone Joint Surg Br 2009; 91(6):835-42.

27. Langton DJ, Sprowson AP, Joyce TJ, et al. Blood metal ion concentrations after hip resurfacing arthroplasty: a comparative study of articular surface replacement and Birmingham hip resurfacing arthroplasties. J Bone Joint Surg Br 2009;91(10):1287-95.

28. Kwon YM, Thomas P, Summer B, et al. Lymphocyte proliferation responses in patients with pseudotumors following metal-on-metal hip resurfacing arthroplasty. J Orthop Res 28(4):444-50.

29. Hartley WT, McAuley JP, Culpepper WJ, et al. Osteonecrosis of the femoral head treated with cementless total hip arthroplasty. J Bone Joint Surg Am 2000;82-A:1408-13.

30. Kantor SG, Huo MH, Huk OL, et al. Cemented total hip arthroplasty in patients with osteonecrosis. A six year minimum follow-up study of second generation cement techniques. J Arthroplasty 1996;11:267-71.

31. Kim YH, Oh SH, Kim JS, et al. Contemporary total hip arthroplasty with and without cement with osteonecrosis of the femoral head. J Bone Joint Surg Am 2003;85-A:675-81.

32. Kim YH, Oh JH, Oh SH. Cementless total hip arthroplasty in patients with osteonecrosis of the femoral head. Clin Orthop Relat Res 1995;320:73-84.

33. Lins RE, Barnes BC, Callaghan JJ, et al. Evaluation of uncemented total hip arthroplasty in patients with avascular necrosis of the femoral head. Clin Orthop Relat Res 1993;297:168-73.

34. Ortiguera CJ, Pulliam IT, Cabanela ME. Total hip arthroplasty for osteonecrosis: matched pair analysis of 188 hips with long-term follow-up. J Arthroplasty 1999;14:21-8.

35. Piston RW, Engh CA, De Carvalho PI, et al. Osteonecrosis of the femoral head treated with total hip arthroplasty without cement. J Bone Joint Surg Am 1994;76:202-14.

36. Stulberg BN, Singer R, Goldner J, et al. Uncemented total hip arthroplasty in osteonecrosis: a 2- to 10- year evaluation. Clin Orthop Relat Res 1997;334:116-23.

37. D'Antonio JA, Capello WN, Manley MT, et al. Hydroxyapatite coated implants. Total hip arthroplasty in the young patient with avascular necrosis. Clin Orthop Relat Res 1997;344:124-38.

38. Mont MA, Seyler TM, Plate JF, et al. Uncemented total hip arthroplasty in young adults with osteonecrosis of the femoral head: a comparative study. J Bone Joint Surg Am 2006;88:104-9.

39. Nich C, Courpied JP, Kerboull M, et al. Charnley-Kerboull total hip arthroplasty for osteonecrosis of the femoral head. A minimal 10-year follow-up study. J Arthroplasty 2006;21:533-40.

40. Seyler TM, Bonutti PM, Shen J, et al. Use of an alumina-on-alumina bearing system in total hip arthroplasty for osteonecrosis of the hip. J Bone Joint Surg Am 2006;88:116-25.

41. Xenakis TA, Beris AE, Malizos KK, et al. Total hip arthroplasty for avascular necrosis and degenerative arthritis of the hip. Clin Orthop Relat Res 1997;341:62-8.

42. Lins RE, Barnes BC, Callaghan JJ, Mair SD, McCollum DE. Evaluation of uncemented total hip arthroplasty in patients with avascular necrosis of the femoral head. Clin Orthop Relat Res 1993; (297):168-73.

43. KimYH, Kim JS, Park JW, Joo JH. Comparison of total hip replacement with and without cement in patients younger than 50 years of age. J Bone Joint Surg [Br] 2011;93-B:449-55.

44. Millar NL, Halai M,McKenna R, McGraw IWW. Miliar LL,Hadidi M. Uncemented Ceramic on ceramic THA in adults with osteonecrosis of femoral head.ORTHOPEDICS November 2010;33(11):795.

45. Augustovski F, Pichon Riviere A, Alcaraz A, et al. Usefulness of ceramic or metal on metal prostheses in total hip replacement [summary]. Report IRR No. 84. Buenos Aires, Argentina: Institute for Clinical Effectiveness and Health Policy (IECS); 2006.

46. Chiu KH, Shen WY, Ko CK, Chan KM. Osteonecrosis of the femoral head treated with cementless total hip arthroplasty. A comparison with other diagnoses. J Arthroplasty 1997;12:683-8.

47. Salvati EA, Cornell CN. Long-term follow-up of total hip replacement in patients with avascular necrosis. Instr Course Lect 1988;37:67-73.

48. Young NL, Cheah D, Waddell JP, Wright JG. Patient characteristics that affect the outcome of total hip arthroplasty: a review. Can J Surg 1998;41:188-95.

49. Alpert B, Waddell JP, Morton J, Bear RA. Cementless total hip arthroplasty in renal transplant patients. Clin Orthop Relat Res 1992;284:164-9.

50. Charles L Nelson, Craig L Israelite, Jonathan P Garino. Total Hip Replacement in Osteonecrosis. Techniques in Orthopaedics 2008; 23(1):74-8.

51. Davis ET, Mckee MD, Waddell JP, Hupel T, Schemitsch EH. Total hip arthroplasty following failure of free vascularized fibular graft. J Bone Joint Surg [Am] 2006;88-A (3):110-5.

52. Berend KR, Gunneson E, Urbaniak JR, Vail TP. Hip arthroplasty after failed free vascularized fibular grafting for osteonecrosis in young patients. J Arthroplasty 2003;18:411-9.

3

Total Hip Arthroplasty Following Acetabular Fractures

P Suryanarayan

Acetabular fractures are complex injuries with the potential for a poor outcome despite application of proper treatment methods.[1-3] Recent studies in the published literature have adequately established the positive association between good long-term result and accuracy of reduction of the articular surface.[2,4]

Despite good anatomic reduction achieved either by operative or nonoperative method of treatment possibility of secondary arthritis of the hip are 30% at 5 years.[4-8]

In spite of this high incidence of secondary arthritis, the value of open reduction and internal fixation of displaced and difficult fractures in restoring acetabular bone stock and minimizing pelvic deformity cannot be over emphasized.[2] Stable osteosynthesis with good congruous articular reduction should be the primary goal in almost all cases of acetabular fractures. Total hip arthroplasty is a salvage for the failure of the initial treatment, painful sequelae or persistent pain and disability. The indications for total hip replacement as a primary method of treatment in acetabular fractures is very limited. It must be emphasized that, one must be well experienced with the various reconstructive methods of osteosynthesis before embarking on a primary total hip for these fractures. Reported complication rates are high and surgery can often be tedious and difficult.

Once symptomatic post-traumatic arthritis has developed, options for salvage are generally, limited to total hip arthroplasty. THR remains the best option for offering mobile, stable hip joint and restore the function. Contributing factors may include an imperfect reduction, osteochondral defects, chon-

drolysis due to articular trauma, avascular necrosis of the femoral head, failed fixations, persistent subluxation etc.[9] Results of total hip arthroplasty following acetabular fractures are inferior to that following primary arthrosis. This is due to the interplay of the other variables peculiar to this clinical situation. Also most of these are consequent to high energy trauma affecting a much younger population group. Thus, age becomes one important variable that deserves serious consideration before a decision of total hip is made.

In view of the principal shortcoming with total hip arthroplasty following an acetabular fracture— namely, the vulnerability to premature failure and the subsequent need for one or more revisions especially in the young male or exceptionally active individuals, potential therapeutic alternatives merit serious consideration.[18] (also ref of Joel Matta). In such patients, one therapeutic alternative is arthrodesis of the hip, which is mainly indicated if there is relative preservation of the osseous architecture of the hip joint. The other criteria to be satisfied for a successful arthrodesis are a normal contralateral hip, normal knees, and an asymptomatic lower back.[19]

Currently, most individuals are reluctant to consider arthrodesis and this is acceptable to fewer and fewer patients, in view of the alteration of gait, function and secondary problems of spine in the long term.[10,11] Thus, despite the published evidence suggesting a higher failure rate in this clinical situation, total hip arthroplasty remains, for most patients a safe, predictable and acceptable alternative. Also, with the use of the newer components with augmented ingrowth potential with lasting stable fixation the results with the current generation of bearings and fixation have improved considerably.

TOTAL HIP ARTHROPLASTY IN ACUTE FRACTURES OF THE ACETABULUM

Consideration of THR in primary situation should be an exception than the rule and osteosynthesis should be primary goal.[26] However, when anatomic reconstruction is not possible due to severe comminution or the anticipated outcome of internal fixation is poor, consideration can be given for a primary hip replacement. The following clinical situations deserve this consideration.

1. More than forty percent cartilage loss either of the head or the socket especially the crucial dome area or the roof arc zone.
2. Articular comminution that makes the anatomic reconstruction impossible.
3. Sectoral bone loss with unstable and persistent dislocation.
4. Elderly low demanded patient with poor bone stock and rigid stable fixation is not possible. Also the medical situation does not allow multiple interventions.
5. Expected poor outcome with osteosynthesis.

There is however no consensus as to the timing of the surgery. Some authors advocate as a primary procedure following the injury. Others recommend a delayed primary intervention after 6 to 10 weeks. The advantage of the latter approach being,

1. The tissue contusion is minimal
2. Some elements of the fracture would have consolidated making the fixation a bit easy.
3. Lesser possibility of ectopic ossification. However, this aspect is not substantiated in the published literature on this subject.

IMPORTANT ISSUES IN SURGERY

1. Uncemented cups are preferable and the results have been more favorable.
2. Ensure stability of the columns since these form the pillars. If there is a fracture or displacement this should be neutralized with additional fixation.

The position of the implants should be planned, so that they do not infringe on the cup placement.

3. Marginal fractures of the posterior wall may be left alone, so long as the residual socket allows at least 70% coverage of the cup. It is necessary to ensure that the postero-superior segment of the socket is stable since this lies in the direct line of stress transfer.
4. In the presence of some displacement, the conventional references for the correct placement of the socket, like the TAL, the margins etc. may not be reliable.
5. Communition of the floor with displacement, would need consideration of bone graft and reconstruction with anti-protrusio devices. If uncemented devices are used it is better to augment the rim fit with additional screws.
6. Guarded and controlled postoperative protocol is necessary.

THR IN OLD ACETABULAR FRACTURES

It is necessary to understand the pathoanatomy of these group of cases and appropriate strategies should be employed for the socket repair. Often they present with prior attempts at osteosynthesis. In our context it is very essential to rule out sepsis. The challenges to get a congruous socket for a cup fixation depends on the type of the fracture. It is important to understand the morphologic changes that have been imposed on the anatomy of acetabulum due to injury. Reconstruction strategies employed are similar to the techniques adopted in revision surgeries.

The fundamental principles in reconstruction are:

1. Restore the center of rotation.
2. Confirm the stability and continuity of the ilio-ischial and the ileopubic columns.
3. Identify if any rotational malunion is present.
4. Ensure adequate host bone cover (70-75%) for the cup.
5. Alter the reconstructive technique based on the features of the given case.

Common pattern of clinical presentations are:

1. Secondary arthritis with previous surgery. Deformation of the socket is minimal. The only issue at times is the presence of implants.

2. Failed internal fixations following acetabular fractures. Loose implants, displacement, persistent subluxation, avascular bone fragments are common. Beware of nonunion of the columns that have been fixed. If still persistent mobility is seen they will need to be fixed. Cases with persistent subluxation/fixed dislocation often show eburnation of the wall and the residual column, further aggravating the bone loss.
3. Displaced acetabular fractures without prior surgeries. Clinical and radiological presentation may vary depending upon the type of fracture.
4. Malunion/nonunion in the roof, columns
5. Complex pelviacetabular fractures with hip dislocation.

Each of these clinical varieties has certain issues that merits considerations in further treatment.

Issues in Planning and Decision Making

1. **Limb-length considerations:** Often the LLD is due to proximal migration of hip joint. Restoration of the hip center will restore the length. In clinical situations with proximal migration of the hemipelvis (associated vertical shear pelvic injury, childhood pelvic injuries, etc.) it may not be possible to restore the LLD. This should be discussed with the patient.
2. **Neurologic status** should be properly assessed and documented.
3. **Choice of prosthesis:** Morphology of fracture, often dictates the choice of the acetabular component. Cemented cups are feasible if the socket deformation is minimal. However, the reported loosening rates for these cups are as high as 15% at 7.5 years, in the Mayo clinic series. Press fit uncemented cups are the implants of choice. Focal areas of bone defect should be filled with morsellised grafts, sectoral bone defects often need bulk femoral head grafts for reconstruction of the defect following which one can either use an uncemented cup or a ring/cage.
4. Proper planning needs a three-dimensional understanding of the altered pelvic anatomy. It is feasible today to create pelvic models with the CT scans. These help immensely in the planning of the reconstructive strategies that may be needed for a given situation. This enables a total rehearsal of the surgery during the planning stage.

Investigations

1. **X-rays:** Anteroposterior, judet views, pelvic inlet and outlet views.
2. **CT scans with reconstruction**
3. **Nerve conduction and velocity studies** to document any neurological involvement
4. **Septic markers:** Complete blood count, erythrocyte sedimentation rate, C-reactive protein.

Surgical Approach

A large number of these cases are associated with posterior defects or lesions. Hence, any approach employed should be expansile and offer good visualization of the posterior strutures for reconstruction. The standard posterior approach is hence the preferred approach. This also enables better appreciation and protection of the sciatic nerve. Should further exposure be needed it can be done easily by one of the following methods:

1. **Additional anterior visualization** by a capsulotomy in front of the gluteus medius.
2. **Trochanteric osteotomy:** This gives an expanded view of the superior and the posterosuperior segments. The disadvantage is the need for refixation. Problems in fixation and union often lead to lurch postoperative.
3. **Trochanteric flip:** This is a modification of the trochanteric osteotomy which involves elevation of a composite sleeve of the vastus lateralis and the gluteus medius as a single sleeve. The function is better preserved.

ACETABULAR RECONSTRUCTION

Surgical Goals

- Stable fixation
- Restore the center of rotation
- Reconstruct the acetabular defects.

Techniques that enable reconstruction of the lost bone are always appealing. No prosthetic construct, today can be considered permanent and thus by restoring the lost bone, one is laying the foundation for the possible future revision. This is especially true in younger individuals undergoing revision. For establishing a treatment approach the clinical situations may be categorized to:

1. Contained (stable) situations, e.g. cavitory defects
2. Uncontained (unstable) situations, e.g. segmental, combined defects. The damage to the columns is considerable and the residual columns may be insufficient to support the new components and will need augmented reconstructions.

CONSIDERATIONS IN SPECIFIC SITUATION

Central Fracture Dislocation

Issues

1. Difficult dislocation
2. Deficiency of floor
3. Proximity of nerve to the posterior margin of trochanter especially in cases with fixed external rotation deformity.

Treatment Plan

1. Restoration of bone deficiency
2. Lateralization of the cup
3. Restore the center of rotation.

Problems with existing implants: It is not mandatory to remove all the implants if they do not come in the way of the reconstruction. Elaborate attempts at removal prolongs the duration of surgery and the danger of further injuring the nerve in the process.

A. **Problems of dislocating the hip:** The situation is similar to the protrusio. The proximal and medial migration, the fractured floor, and the scarring in the socket may make the dislocation very difficult. Additional extensile measures need to be employed. Also there is often constriction of the mouth of the cup due to bone formation or the scarring. This is again an impediment to the dislocation. Attempts at forced rotation and dislocation increases the chances of fractures of the shaft. Complete mobilization, capsulotomy and lateral dislocation are the key elements.

B. **Avoiding nerve injuries:** The medial migration decreases the distance between the posterior trochanteric margin and the nerve, with potential for injury. Some possible preventive strategies are:
   - Palpate the nerve or identify the perineural fat and the nerve
   - Do not dissect to remove the posterior implants
   - Dissect close to the bone and reflect the capsulomuscular structures as a single layer. This in turn protects the nerve.

C. **Correction of the medialization:** In pure central fracture dislocations, the columns are often intact. These enable a good peripheral rim fixation of the socket. The lateralization is achieved with grafting of the floor defect with morsellised grafts compacted well. Ensure that the cup is seated well. Some medialization in this regard is useful. Up to 3 to 4 mm of medialization to Kohler's line is acceptable. The stability can be further augmented with the use of screws. Hemispherical Press fit devices with various surface treatments that enable bone ingrowth have given the best results. The survival of these reconstructions with end point as revision for aseptic loosening exceeds 93% in minimum 10 to 15 years follow-ups.[23]

The prerequisites are:

1. Intact supporting columns
2. Adequate host bone contact - minimum 70%

It is the fit between the columns (anteroposterior) that determines the stability.

If the surface contact is between 50 to 70%, it is categorized as being partially supportive. Though not the ideal situation press fit cups may still be used in this situation if the deficiency is not predominantly in the vital areas, like in some segmental defects.

Surface contact less than 50% is inadequate and will require other options. If there are associated posterior wall or column fractures compromising the rim fixation and stability, the situation might need the use of support rings or a cage. Beware to avoid excessive laterization with this technique.

Posterior Fracture Dislocation

These are uncontained defects which almost always requires some augmentation. Often there is deficiency of the posterior cover. The common mistake is fixing the cups in retroversion.

Issues

1. Proximal migration of the hip center
2. Persistent posterior subluxation
3. Posterior deficiency and an unsupported socket defect.
4. Posterior column nonunion.

Treatment Plan

A. Restore the hip center
B. Bone graft to convert the uncontained defect to a contained one.
C. Stable fixation of the socket device.

Often the posterior wall fragments are malunited at a more proximal level. It is permissible to shift the center of rotation high up to 1 cm in these situations and place the cup rigidly against the native bone. Results of a high hip center up to 1 to 1.5 cm have been good without any long-term consequence. Identify some native landmarks of original acetabulum like ligamentum transversarium and cotyloid fossa, during the preoperative planning which serves as a good template and a starting point in the reconstruction. In previously nonoperated cases the patients own femoral head could be used for the defect reconstruction. If there is residual mobility of columns, additional osteosynthesis will be required. Place the posterior column implants away from the wall and more medially so that it does not come in the way of the cup fixation. Oblong cups and large cups though attractive, are better avoided since the results in the long term are not encouraging.

PRINCIPLES IN THE USE OF BLOCK ALLOGRAFTS FOR RECONSTRUCTION

Block allografts (femoral head, distal femur, acetabulum). Though they have been an excellent option for major reconstructions, there have been some concerns with regard to their long-term behavior. This is due to the poor revascularization of the bulk graft leading to failure, resorption and late collapse.[21]

Some important considerations in their use are:
a. Should be adequately protected.
b. Using autografts at the margins is recommended.
c. Should be big enough to avoid late revascularization and collapse.
d. Bulk grafts protected by support rings and cages have performed better
e. It is also useful to orient the graft along the stress lines while fixing. This also protects the grafts from collapse.[24]

Reconstruction Rings and Cages

There are a variety of rings and cages used. Principally they are anchored and fixed solidly to the remaining cortical bone in the ileum, ischium or pubis. A polyethylene cup is then cemented into the ring or cage. Commonly used devices are Muller roof reinforcement ring, Burch Schneider cage, ring with hook, etc.

Features and Necessary Aspects

a. Act as anti-protrusio devices and act as a conduit for force transmission.
b. Transmit the body load to the columns.
c. Protect the grafts behind them from over load.
d. The cage and hook devices help in restoring the hip rotation center.
e. It is important to realize that these are non-integrating devices and only works as a mechanical bridges and hence exposed to stress and strains of motion.
f. Preferably chosen implant should be precontoured to acetabular shape and further contouring better avoided.
g. If teardrop area is intact cages, with hooks are preferred as this minimizes the dissection and these devices are often self-contouring.
h. If cages with ischial extension is chosen it is ideal to impact the ischial fins into the bone mass as

in vitro study shows that fixation of fin over the surface of ischium by screws is often inadequate and fails.

i. The proximal screw of ileal segment should be in direction of stress namely towards the sacroiliac joint. This avoids stress deformation and fatigue failure.

They are very useful in cases with:

a. Medial wall defect (protrusio)
b. Segmental defects reconstructed with grafts
c. Osteoporotic bones.

Reconstruction of superior lateral defects—restoration of the hip center is facilitated by the combined use of grafts and cages or ring with hook.

It is worth mention here that in uncemented cup fixation on ring or cage; both should be in proper version. In cemented cup fixation on ring or cage some version can be adjusted by cup. This is important to take care in posterior wall deficiencies as there may be chances of retroversion. Large heads are of course useful in preventing the dislocation in any of these situations.

COMPLEX SITUATIONS

These are unusual situations. Often they are combined pelviacetabular injuries. The treatment plan in these cases need to be individualized. Total hip replacement in these situations can be difficult since it involves identification and neutralization of malunion/nonunions of the vital segments of the periacetabular area. The basic principles of reconstruction are:

1. Stability of posterior column.
2. Integrity of sacroiliac joint and confirm pelvi femoral continuity along the lines of stress transfer. It must be pointed out that it is not necessary to internally fix the forepelvic components of the injury like the ileal wing fractures, since they do not contribute to the stress transfer.
3. At least minimum support to posterosuperior area for stable fixation of cup.
4. Postoperatively the rehabilitation should be altered appropriately.

COMPLICATIONS

As problems of difficulty in dislocation, postoperative dislocation, nerve injuries are always there. Apart from that chances of heterotropic ossification, higher chances of bleeding and infection are also there. Chances of heterotropic ossification can be minimized by better soft tissue handling, postoperative radiation or indomethacin used as a NSAID.

FUTURE

For the years uncemented devices worked well. Tantalum augments and prenavigated innominate bones could be more in use as revision cases in total hip replaced patients in prior acetabular fractures will increase along with increase in life expectancy and technologies.

REFERENCES

1. Carnesale PG, Stewart MJ, Barnes SN. Acetabular disruption and central fracture-dislocation of the hip. A long-term study. J Bone Joint Surg Am 1975;57:1054-9.
2. Letournel E. The treatment of acetabular fractures through the ilioinguinal approach. Clin Orthop 1993;292:62-76.
3. Matta JM, Merritt PO. Displaced acetabular fractures. Clin Orthop 1988;230:83-97.
4. Matta JM. Fractures of the acetabulum: accuracy of reduction and clinical results in patients managed operatively within three weeks after the injury. J Bone Joint Surg Am 1996;78:1632-45.
5. Mayo KA. Open reduction and internal fixation of fractures of the acetabulum. Results in 163 fractures. Clin Orthop 1994;305:31-7.
6. Wright R, Barrett K, Christie MJ, Johnson KD. Acetabular fractures: long-term follow-up of open reduction and internal fixation. J Orthop Trauma 1994;8:397-403.
7. Pennal GF, Davidson J, Garside H, Plewes J. Results of treatment of acetabular fractures. Clin Orthop 1980;151:115-23.
8. Ragnarsson B, Mjoberg B. Arthrosis after surgically treated acetabular fractures. A retrospective study of 60 cases. Acta Orthop Scand 1992;63:511-4.

9. Jimenez ML, Tile M, Schenk RS. Total hip replacement after acetabular fracture. Orthop Clin North Am 1997;28:435-46.

10. Greiss ME, Thomas RJ, Freeman MA. Sequelae of arthrodesis of the hip. JR Soc Med 1980;73:497-500.

11. Missiuna PC, Dewar RD. Long-term sequelae of hip fusion surgery. Orthop Trans 1988;12:672.

12. Joly JM, Mears DC, Skura DS. Total hip arthroplasty following failed acetabular fracture open reduction/internal fixation. Read at the Annual Meeting of the American Academy of Orthopaedic Surgeons 1993 Feb 19; San Francisco, CA.

13. Karpik K, Mears DC, Hardy SL. Total hip arthroplasty for posttraumatic arthritis following acetabular fracture. Read at the Annual Meeting of the Orthopaedic Trauma Association 1995 Oct 1; Tampa, FL.

14. Karpos PA, Christie MJ, Chenger JD. Total hip arthroplasty following acetabular fracture: the effect of prior open reduction, internal fixation. Orthop Trans 1993;17:589.

15. Rogan IM, Weber FA, Solomon L. Total hip replacement following fracture dislocation of the acetabulum. In Proceedings of the South African Orthopaedic Association. J Bone Joint Surg Br 1979;61:252.

16. Romness DW, Lewallen DG. Total hip arthroplasty after fracture of the acetabulum. Long-term results. J Bone Joint Surg Br 1990;72:761-4.

17. Stauffer RN. Ten-year follow-up study of total hip replacement. J Bone Joint Surg Am 1982;64:983-90.

18. Weber M, Berry DJ, Harmsen WS. Total hip arthroplasty after operative treatment of an acetabular fracture. J Bone Joint Surg Am 1998;80:1295-1305.

19. Mont MA, Maar DC, Krackow KA, Jacobs MA, Jones LC, Hungerford DS. Total hip replacement without cement for non-inflammatory osteoarthrosis in patients who are less than forty-five years old. J Bone and Joint Surg 1993;75-A:740-51.

20. Callaghan JJ, McBeath: Arthrodesis. In the Adult Hip, pp. 749-759. Edited by JJ Callaghan, AG Rosenberg, and HE Rubash. Philadelphia, Lippincott-Raven, 1998.

21. Harris WH. The problem is osteolysis. Clin Orthop 1995;311:46-53.

22. D'Antonio J, McCarthy JC, Barger WL, et al. Classification of femoral abnormalities in total hip arthroplasty. Clin orthop 1993;296:133-9.

23. Cuckler JM. Management strategies for acetabular defects in revision total hip arthroplasty. J Arthroplasty 2002;14(4 suppl 1):153-6.

24. Head WC, Malinin TI. Results of onlay allografts. Clin Orthop 2000;371:108-12.

25. Thien TM, Welten ML, Verdonschot N, et al. Acetabular revision with impacted freeze dried cancellous bone chips and a cemented cup: a report of seven cases at 5 to 9 years follow-up. J Arthroplasty 2001;16:666-70.

26. Primary Total hip arthroplasty after acetabular fractures. Dana Mears, Journal of Bone and Joint Surgery 2000.pp.1328-53.

4 | Total Hip Replacement for Failed Trochanteric Fractures

C Thakkar

Internal fixation of Intertrochanteric fracture with various devices is a standard treatment. At one time dynamic hip screw (DHS) was preferred implant[1] but today various intramedullary devices are preferred over DHS as they are supposed to be load sharing devices allowing early mobilization even in presence of communition and osteoporosis. In spite of best of efforts, certain number of patients still end up with failure of fixation[2,3] due to various reasons like poor bone quality, suboptimal reduction of fracture, and suboptimal implant placement. This would result in malnonunion in varus and external rotation, causing pain, shortening and limp while walking. There could be implant penetration in the joint leading to secondary arthrosis.

The decision to manage the failure either by re-osteosynthesis or replacement arthroplasty depends on; the age of the patient, bone quality, available bone for reconstruction, presence of joint penetration with associated acetabular changes, medical comorbidities affecting longevity and experience of treating surgeon.[4-6]

If one decides to consider replacement as treatment option, the choice between hemireplacement and total replacement would depend on status of articular cartilage of the acetabulum and the age of the patient. In patients with life-expectancy less than 7 years with good acetabulum, one may offer hemireplacement.[7]

The choice between cemented or uncemented replacement will depend again on age of the patient, quality of bone according to Dorr,[8] surgeon experience and preference and finally the cost.

PREOPERATIVE PLANNING

Following issues need to be addressed while planning the surgery:
- Implant removal, whether before or after dislocation
- Filling/bypassing screw holes
- Management of broken screws/drill bits
- Greater trochanter
- Lesser trochanter
- Proximal bone loss.

These are major surgeries carrying high morbidity. It is essential to obtain physician fitness. The anesthetist must be informed about prolonged duration of surgery, requirement for hypotensive measures to prevent excessive blood loss, need for multiple blood transfusions during the surgery and postoperative intensive care unit observation.

The choice of anesthesia is left to the anesthetist, but we prefer epidural anesthesia supplemented with general anesthesia with possibility of adequate hypotension to ease dissection through inflamed tissues.

The following points must be considered while templeting the femur:
- Look for broken intramedullary nail, screws and drill bits, which may pose problem of removal unless appropriate instruments are kept handy.
- The medullary canal may be wide due to osteoporosis related to age and disuse; requiring implant of large size or consideration for cemented implant.
- The proximal end of canal may be closed with sclerotic bone, which may require to be penetrated with sharp awl or 4.5 drill.

- The medial and posteromedial proximal femur may be deficient requiring calcar replacement prosthesis[3] or use of structural bone graft.
- The lateral view of the femoral shaft may reveal excessive anterior bowing. In this situation long revision prosthesis with straight stem may lead to iatrogenic fracture at the tip of the prosthesis or anterior cortex impingement causing pain.

Careful attention must be paid to the status of greater trochanter. Because the success and longevity of the implanted prosthesis will depend upon the management of abductor mechanism. The greater trochanter may have migrated proximally, requiring considerable dissection to bring it back to its original position. It may be fragmented posing challenge to fix it to the prosthesis or it may be osteoporotic requiring attention to postoperative mobilization to avoid wire cut out. In cases of malunion, the trochanter may overhang the entry point of the femoral prosthesis, forcing the implant in varus position.

Implant selection: We prefer noncemented revision stem if the expected longevity is more than 7 to 10 years. We generally prefer porous coated titanium stem-like solution (J and J), this monobloc implant has predominently metaphysial fit and has option of calcar replacement if the proximal medial bone is deficient. This stem has an advantage over the Wagner stem, which we used in past, in that, it has anatomic bow of femur and hence there is less chance of tip of the stem impinging against anterior cortex causing pain or in some instances causing iatrogenic fracture on the table. It is essential that the femoral implant length is two cortical diameter beyond the last screw hole to prevent stress fracture in the postoperative period.[9,10]

One can also choose from other available stem options which allow distal locking, like Aesculap Bicontact prosthesis. We are not in favor of using modular stem like S-Rom as it has no advantage over monobloc stems and are also more expensive.

The reason for not selecting cemented femoral stem is that it becomes difficult to pressurize bone cement due to presence of screw holes. One may block the lateral holes tempoprarily by inserting the screws in these holes till the cement sets, but the medial cortical holes still pose is a problem. If we do opt for cemented stem option, our choice is polished double taper stem of Exeter (Howmedica).

Total hip replacement versus bipolar: If the acetabular articulation is eroded due to penetrating implant or is arthritic, there is no choice but to resurface it. But if the acetabular cartilage is good and if the patient has limited activity or lifespan, then we would consider bipolar replacement. The advantage of bipolar replacement is reduction in the surgical morbidity as well as being of anatomic head size, there is less possibility of dislocation.

SURGICAL TECHNIQUE

We prefer posterolateral approach because of our familiarity with the same.

Following issues need to be addressed:

Removal of implant: If the implant has not penetrated the joint, we prefer to dislocate the hip joint before implant removal. This reduces the risk of fracture through the bone weakened by void created after implant removal.

If one encounters broken screws or drill bits in the shaft, it is imperative to remove these, else they may impinge on the femoral stem and if one is using a titanium stem, the stainless screw, which are normally used, may lead to galvanic corrosion.

Bone grafts/bone augments: In some cases, when, there is proximal medial void and the canal is not wide enough to accept calcar replacement Solution prosthesis, which comes in diameter 15 and above, we harvest bone graft from calcar region of the proximal fragment and use is as a graft in the void. We have a large experience of this technique in replacement in cases of fresh intertrochanteric fracture. The graft is usually wedged between the medial surface of the femoral prosthesis and endosteal surface of the medial femoral cortex. Rarely we may use an interfragmetary screw to fix this bone graft.

Restoration of limb length is of paramount importance, because this would add to the comfort and confidence of geriatric patient, who may have associated neurological conditions, making him unstable. Preoperative templeting will help in correct placement of femoral implant and would suggest the need of bone graft for reconstruction of void, if any.

Management of greater trochanter: Restoration of abductor tension is most important step in this complex surgery. It prevents chances of immediate and late dislocations and prevents abductor lurch. In situations where the greater trochanter is migrated proximally and is difficult to adequately bring it down, gap may remain between the trochanter and the shaft, this may need to be filled up. We use autograft from the femoral head, which is shaped in the form of bone block and is inserted in the gap and the greater trochanter is then wired to the shaft, thus locking the graft in position.

We prefer multiple stainless steel wireloops to fix the trochanter to the femoral shaft. We have no experience with use of cable. Comminution, osteoporosis, small size and proximal migration makes fixation of trochanter far more demanding than fixation of the femoral implant. In spite of various techniques, patients must be warned of residual problems of greater trochanter.

To prevent complication of iatrogenic fracture intraoperatively, use of C-arm while reaming and prosthesis insertion is a very good idea.[11] In an unfortunate eventuality of its occurrence, one may need to open the fracture site and use locking plates to fix the fracture. This increases the surgical morbidity and delays the mobilization.

Postoperative protocol: Our general protocol is to put the patients on calf compression pump for prevention of DVT. Unless specifically suggested by the attending physician, we do not routinely use low molecular weight heparin in our patients.

The mobilization schedule will depend on the previously described factors of age, general condition, bone quality and quality of trochanteric stabilization.

Preoperatively all the patients are trained in static exercises of stance group of muscles, deep breathing exercises. Since majority of patients are reasonably well trained in partial weight-bearing after their index fixation surgery, to follow the same with fewer modification is not difficult.

We prefer partial weight bearing of 10% in the first two weeks, gradually increasing to 25% in the third week and increasing by 25% on weekly basis. Majority of the patients achieve full weight-bearing with support by end of 6 to 8 weeks. Many retain walking support for rest of their life, while some discard it, if they feel confident enough. This decision is taken by the operating surgeon in consultation with the patient.

RESULTS IN LITERATURE

Author	Patients	FU	Result
Mariani and Rand[12]	9	6.6 years	All OK
Stoffelen[13]	7		5 Excellent to good
Melhoff[14]	13	34 months	5 Good, 3 dislocations
Haiduykewych and Berry[3]	60	5 years	7 years survivorship 100%

REFERENCES

1. Doppelt SH. The sliding compression screw: Today's best answer for stabilization of intertrochanteric hip fractures. Orthop Clin North Am 1980;11:507-23.
2. Eschenroeder HC Jr, Krackow KA. Late onset femoral stress fracture associated with extruded cement following hip arthroplasty: A case report. Clin Orthop 1988;236:210-3.
3. Functional outcome of fracture neck of femur treated with total hip replacement versus bipolar arthroplasty in a South Asian population: Archives of Truama and orthopaedic surgery. volume 126. Number 8/ October, 2006.
4. Haentjens P, Casteleyn PP, Opdecam P. Hip arthroplasty for failed internal fixation of intertrochanteric and subtrochanteric fractures in the elderly patient. Arch Orthop Trauma Surg 1994;113:222-7.
5. Haidukewych GJ, Berry DJ. Hip arthroplasty for salvage of failed intertrochanteric hip fractures. J Bone Joint Surg Am 2003;85:899-905.
6. Kim Y-H, Oh J-H, Koh Y-G. Salvage of neglected unstable intertrochanteric fracture with cementless porous-coated hemiarthroplasty. Clin Orthop 1992; 277:182-7.
7. Kyle RF, Cabanela ME, Russell TA, Swiontkowski MF, Winquist RA, Zuckerman JD, Schmidt AH, Koval KJ. Fractures of the proximal part of the femur. Instr Course Lect 1995;44:227-53.

8. Thakur RR, Desmukh Ajit J, Goyal A, Ranawat AS, Rasquinha VJ, Rodriguez JA. Management of failed trochanteric fracture fixation with cementless modular hip anthroplasty using a distally fixing stem. Article in press, Journal of Anthroplasty.

9. Mariani EM, Rand JA. Nonunion of intertrochanteric fractures of the femur following open reduction and internal fixation: Results of second attempts to gain union. Clin Orthop 1987;218:81-9.

10. Mehlhoff T, Landon GC, Tullos HS. Total hip arthroplasty following failed internal fixation of hip fractures. Clin Orthop. 1991;269:32-7.

11. Optimising results of total hip arthroplasty AAOS Instructional lecture course. XXX1V St Louis: Mosby 1985. pp. 401-4.

12. Patterson BM, Salvati EA, Huo MH. Total hip arthroplasty for complications of intertrochanteric fracture: A technical note. J Bone Joint Surg Am. 1990;72:776-7.

13. Stoffelen D, Haentjens P, Reynders P, et al. Hip arthroplasty for failed internal fixation of intertrochanteric and subtrochanteric fractures in the elderly patient. Acta Orthop Belg. 1994;60:135-9.

14. Tabsh I, Waddell JP, Morton J. Total hip arthroplasty for complications of proximal femoral fractures. J Orthop Trauma. 1997;11:166-9.

TOTAL HIP REPLACEMENT FOR FAILED TROCHANTERIC FRACTURES

5 | Total Hip Replacement in Protrusio Acetabuli

Anil Mehtani

PROTRUSIO ACETABULI

Protrusio acetabuli is the inward displacement of the acetabular floor into the pelvic basin, resulting in deepening of socket with associated medial migration of the femoral head.

Also referred as *Arthrokatadysis*—a Greek word meaning subsidence of joint.

TYPES/ETIOLOGY

Essentially it is of two types:

1. *Primary protrusio*: It is also commonly referred as "Otto pelvis", as the condition was first described by Adolf William Otto, a German pathologist on a desiccated specimen from Natural History Museum of Berslau in Poland.

   This rare entity is an idiopathic variety of Protrusio that happens *de novo* without any identifiable underlying pathology. The condition is characteristically bilateral, familial and has marked female preponderance.

   There is also a racial influence as there is increased incidence in Bantu women (an African tribe).

   The pathology develops during childhood or adolescence but more often the condition remains unrecognized for a long time until degenerative arthritis develops.

2. *Secondary protrusio:* This is the usual and the common variety of protrusio that may result from pathologies of diverse origin (Figures 1 to 6). Any disease process that weakens or destroys the bone substrate locally or globally will allow the femoral head to migrate axially (i.e. supero-medially) under the load close to the line of joint reaction forces.

Common causes of secondary protrusio are:

Infection	Tuberculosis Pyogenic – *Staphylococcus, Streptococcus Gonococcus, Echinococcus, Syphilis*, etc.
Inflammation	Rheumatoid arthritis Ankylosing spondylitis Idiopathic chondrolysis Psoriatic arthritis
Metabolic	Osteomalacia Paget's disease Hyperparathyroidism
Genetic disorders	Osteogenesis imperfecta Ehlers-Danlos syndrome Marfan's syndrome Sickle cell disease
Neoplastic	Secondaries Neurofibromatosis Hemangioma
Trauma	Acetabular fractures
Others	Sequelae of hemiarthroplasty Failed total hip arthroplasty Radiation induced osteonecrosis

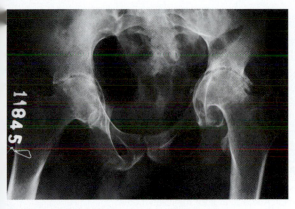

Figure 1: Rheumatoid arthritis

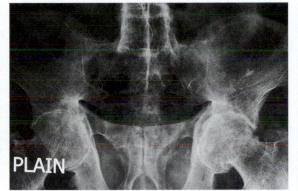

Figure 2: Ankylosing spondylitis

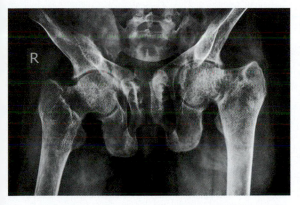

Figure 3: Osteomalacia—Trifoliate pelvis

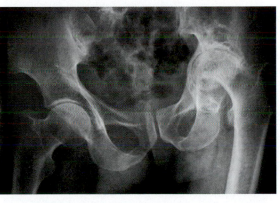

Figure 4: Healed central fracture dislocation

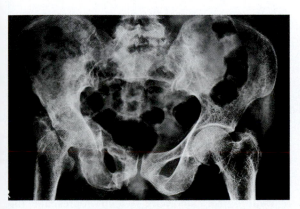

Figure 5: Active tuberculosis

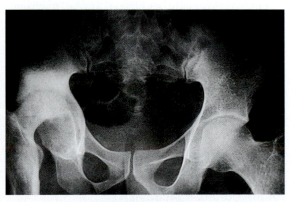

Figure 6: Healed tuberculosis

Figures 1 to 6: Radiographs showing protrusio acetabuli due to various etiologies

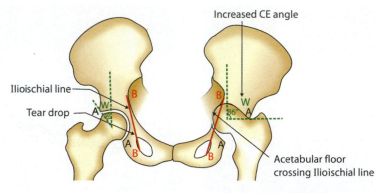

Figure 7: Diagnosis of protrusio acetabuli. Acetabular floor migrates medial to ilioischial line and increased CE angle on left side

CLINICAL FEATURES

The clinical diagnosis of protrusio is often over-looked, especially in younger patients until secondary degenerative changes supervene.

The clinical features of protrusio fall into three categories:

a. *Symptoms due to anatomical abnormality (deepening of socket):* Typically there is increased stiffness and lack of hip flexibility rather than pain. Sitting cross legged may sometimes be the first difficulty coming to notice.

b. *Symptoms due to secondary osteoarthritis:* Pain and limp appear as osteoarthritis supervenes. All movements become progressively painful and limited, especially abduction as the trochanter starts impinging on the superior acetabular margin. A better arc of flexion is often preserved. There may be increased lumbar lordosis due to flexion deformity of the hip. The hip tends to become increasingly stiff leading even to ankylosis. Rectal examination reveals a globular mass on the lateral rectal wall in severe protrusio.

c. *Symptoms due to causative disease:* For examples s/s of rheumatoid arthritis, tuberculosis, osteomalacia, etc.

RADIOLOGICAL ASSESSMENT

The first diagnosis of protrusio is often an incidental finding on radiological assessment for some other pathology rather than for protrusio itself.

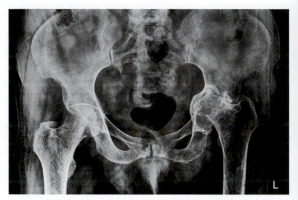

Figure 8: Radiograph showing protrusio in healed tuberculosis left hip. Acetabular floor crossing ilioischial line

A well-centered standard anteroposterior view of the pelvis with both hips is simply required to clinch the diagnosis of protrusio. The classical diagnostic criterion is that 'the outline of the floor of the acetabulum protrudes beyond the ilioischial line (Kohler's line)'.

The ilioischial line extends from the pelvic border of the ilium at the sciatic notch to the medial border of the body of ischium at the obturator foramen, almost brushing the medial acetabular wall on its course (Figures 7 and 8). This is just a radiological landmark which represents the quadrilateral plate of the acetabulum that projects over the medial acetabular wall due to tangency of X-ray beam.[8,18]

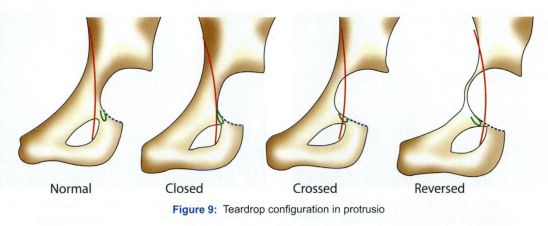

Normal   Closed   Crossed   Reversed

Figure 9: Teardrop configuration in protrusio

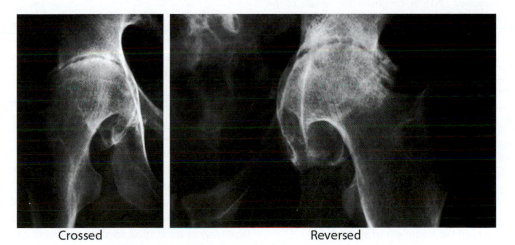

Crossed   Reversed

Figure 10: Radiograph showing teardrop crossed and reversed

Apart from the ilioischial line other commonly used radiological parameters to assess protrusio on AP view of the pelvis with both hips are:

Teardrop Configuration

The teardrop is an 'U'shaped figure located at the inferomedial part of the acetabulum just superior to the obturator foramen (Figures 9 and 10). This is the most accurate anatomical as well as radiological landmark representing the integrity of the acetabulum.[8]

The straight medial limb of the U figure is the pelvic side and represents the inner portion of the acetabular wall and the curved lateral limb is the outer acetabular wall on the articulating side. The lateral limb is dynamic and is altered in a pathological process of the acetabulum. The dynamic lateral limb of U migrates medially in progression of protrusio manifesting on radiographs first as closing then crossing and finally even a reversal of teardrop (Figures 9 and 10).[8,18,30]

Center Edge Angle of Wiberg (CE angle) (Normal Value = 25-40°)

This is the angle between the perpendicular through the femoral head center and the upper and outer margin of acetabulum (Figure 7). It may be increased

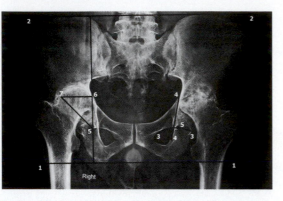

Figure 11: X-ray pelvis showing method of locating anatomical position of acetabulum by Ranawat's method. Two horizontal lines at the levels of iliac crests (2-2) and ischial tuberosities (1-1) to determine the height of the pelvis are marked. On left side, a point (5) is marked 5 mm lateral to the intersection of ilioischial (4-4) and Shenton's line (3-3). On right side, similar point (5) is also marked. A perpendicular through this point is drawn joining the two horizontal lines. A second point (6) is located on the perpendicular line superior to point (5) at a distance equal to one-fifth of the pelvic height. A second perpendicular is drawn laterally from point (6) to point (7) equal to the distance between (5) and (6). Join points (5) and (7). The vertical line 5-6 is the height of the acetabulum, 6-7 is the roof of the acetabulum and the hypotenuse of the isosceles triangle (5-7) is the diameter of the acetabulum

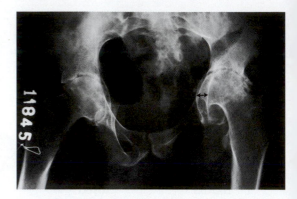

Figure 12: Radiograph showing the measurement of protrusio between ilio-ischial and acetabular line

to more than 40° in protrusio. However, it does not help in planning the treatment of protrusio.[36]

Ranawat's Method of Drawing of Isosceles Triangles

This method is of a good academic value and may be useful for the anatomical location of the hip center in cases with bilateral hip involvement where the architecture, anatomy and configuration of acetabulum are totally lost[26] (Figure 11).

Judet views of the pelvis should also be assessed in cases of Protrusio due to acetabular fractures.

A CT scan with 3D reconstruction is almost obligatory in cases of protrusio following acetabular fractures and destructive lesions of acetabulum such as tubercular infection etc., so as to get an elaborate assessment of the medial wall defect, the integrity of the anterior and posterior walls (rims) as well as the columns of acetabulum. This would help in

preoperative planning, especially in assessing the ability to achieve secure fixation of the socket and to anticipate the need of special rings or cages, etc. to reinforce the acetabulum.

MEASUREMENT AND GRADING OF PROTRUSIO

The protrusio often has a tendency to progress, more so in rheumatoid arthritis. Corticosteroids and the active disease have been implicated as risk factors for the progression in rheumatoid arthritis.[12]

The ilioischial line is more commonly used landmark to measure the amount of protrusion.[15] The Protrusio is quantified as the transverse distance in millimetres of acetabular dome protruding medially across the ilioischial line (Kohler's line) (Figure 12).

However, Sotelo-Garza and Charnley[35] graded the deformity in Protrusio by using the iliopectineal line as the reference (Figure 13). The distance between the upper margin of the superior pubic ramus extending on to the rim of the true pelvis and the outline of the acetabulum protruding into the pelvis was measured and graded accordingly into three grades:

- Grade I (mild Protrusio) 1 to 5 mm
- Grade II (moderate Protrusio) 6 to 15 mm and
- Grade III (severe Protrusio) more than 15 mm.

In a progressive protrusio, usually, the progression is both medial as well as superior.[15] Superior progression can be assessed on serial roentgenograms by measuring the distance between iliac crest and the roof of the acetabulum.[12]

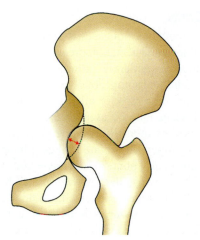

Figure 13: Grading by Sotelo-Garza and Charnley

TOTAL HIP ARTHROPLASTY IN PROTRUSIO

Total hip arthroplasty remains the procedure of choice for protrusio acetabuli in skeletally mature patients with painful and stiff hip having severe degenerative arthritis. However, in a younger patient under 40 years of age and with no degenerative changes, apart from physiotherapy, a valgus intertrochanteric osteotomy may sometimes be considered.

Issues and Principles of Reconstruction by Total Hip Arthroplasty

Reconstruction in protrusio by THA could be demanding because of the deformities, long standing soft tissue contractures, stiffness and limb shortening. However, the main technical issues are the bony inadequacy in the medial acetabular floor and an altered center of rotation of the hip to an abnormal medial position.

The importance of restoration of the original biomechanics and normalization of the hip center has been emphasized in the primary acetabular reconstruction. Iatrogenic acetabular protrusio (over-reaming and medialization of socket) during total hip replacement has been associated with early acetabular loosening.[20] Ranawat and Dorr et al.[26] reported accelerated component loosening on long-term follow-up when the center of rotation of the hip is not

corrected to within 10 mm of the anatomical extent. Other studies have also documented a similar view.[1-6]

The principles and objectives of reconstruction of protrusio by THR are thus underline:
a. Re-enforcement of the deficient medial acetabular wall to prevent a further progression of protrusio and medial migration of the cup.
b. Restoration of the hip center to the near anatomical position by implanting the acetabular component from an abnormal medial position to a near normal lateral position so as to achieve normal biomechanics and a long-term survival of the reconstruction.

Several techniques have been used and reported to achieve these goals which include reconstruction of acetabulum with:
1. Extra amount of bone cement and a cemented socket.[35]
2. Bone grafts with a cemented socket.[6,14,21,25]
3. Metal reinforcements (protrusio rings, cages or wire mesh), with a cemented socket, either with or without bone grafts.[17,22]
4. Bone grafts with a cementless socket.[9]

Sotelo-Garza and Charnley,[35] in the initial reports of reconstruction for protrusio, used extra amount of bone cement for augmentation with a cemented socket. They reported satisfactory results on long-term follow-up and concluded that "there was no difference in the successful results whether a bone graft or cement alone had been used". But subsequent reports in the literature, in total contradiction to the above observations, documented a progression of protrusio with early component loosening when cement fixation alone is used without medially placed bone grafts.[21] Later a study (Hirst and Murphy[14] et al. 1987), from Charnley Center for Hip Replacement itself, recommended the use of impacted medial bone grafts in the form of wafers of 2 mm from the sacrificed femoral head with flanged cemented sockets. They observed that these grafts become incorporated into the floor of the acetabulum and also protect the thin medial acetabular wall from "thermal effects of polymerization" of the poly-methylmethaacrylate. Garcia-Cimbrelo et al.[5] reported "better results after Low Friction Arthroplasty in hips with moderate and severe protrusions reconstructed with bone grafting than in hips with mild protrusion which were not grafted". McCollum et al.[21] concluded that metallic restraining devices (like rings, cages or wire mesh) should be supplemented with bone grafts to provide a lasting support. These mechanical devices without bone grafts may eventually fail when used alone because of the differences in the modulus of elasticity between the metal and bone and protrusion of the acetabulum may progress. Unacceptable long-term results were reported by Jasty and Harris[16] when cement and wire mesh alone was used. The literature also suggests that both cemented and uncemented cups function well clinically; however, uncemented cups demonstrate a lesser rate of loosening than cemented cups in long-term.[9]

From the evidences in the literature it follows that for a reconstruction of protrusio by total hip arthroplasty the technique that is uniformly successful and durable entails:

i. Compacted bone grafting medially to reinforce and repair the weak medial wall and lateralize the socket to the anatomical near normal position. This shall also restore normal length and shift the weight bearing stresses peripherally under the acetabular roof.[31]

ii. A cemented or an uncemented socket: Presently, the uncemented sockets are preferred and are more popular as they give consistently good radiological and clinical results.[9]

If the medial defect is large, one of the restraining metal devices (e.g. protrusio rings, protrusio cages or a metallic mesh) may be used in addition to the bone graft so that the cup and the cement mass will be stabilized during the period of healing and incorporation of the graft. These metal devices help in distributing the forces at the periphery of the acetabulum and prevent further progression of the protrusio and medial migration of the cup. However, if the peripheral rim is intact, which often is the case in protrusio, an uncemented hemispherical porous coated cup is still a better choice. In these cases the medial defect can be blocked by a wire mesh or large bone graft wafers before impacting the morsellized bone grafts.

Bone Grafts

Often autogenous bone grafts from the sacrificed femoral head and acetabular reamings are sufficient for a mild-to-moderate protrusion. For a severe defect, additional autogenous corticocancellous bone grafts from iliac crest or allografts from preserved femoral heads may be used. These grafts could be in the form of morsellized bone grafts of 1-3 mm size[21] prepared with a bone mill or a bone nibbler, thin wafers of about 2 mm removed from the femoral head by oscillating saw[14] or may be a single bulk graft.[13] Compacted morsellized bone grafts are a better method as they rapidly heal and remodel. There is complete consolidation, revascularization and incorporation of the graft with viable bone marrow by 48 weeks.[33] By contrast, bulk (structural) grafts show high failure rates and are at a risk of mechanical weakening during creeping substitution and they may fail to provide a strong buttress to the medial wall at the time when it is needed.[33] In cases of medial wall defect, grafts in the form of thin wafers may be more useful to block the defect. Also they offer resistance during introduction of the cement and cement pressurization.[14]

The bone grafts, apart from reducing thermal damage to medial acetabular wall and lateralizing the cup, are a biological solution for the replacement of the deficient bone in the medial acetabulum. These grafts ultimately get incorporated and remodelled and consequently leave a much more satisfactory bed for any future revisions.[14] Also there is general consensus that medial bone grafting is more likely to arrest the progression of protrusio than acetabular reconstruction without bone graft.[7, 25]

Preoperative Planning

Few essentials are:
1. AP radiograph of pelvis with both hips
   a. To evaluate medial and superior extent of protrusio.
   b. To locate the anatomical center of rotation
   c. To template the acetabular component at the anatomical center of rotation. If contemplating a cementless cup, a large cup is required. This

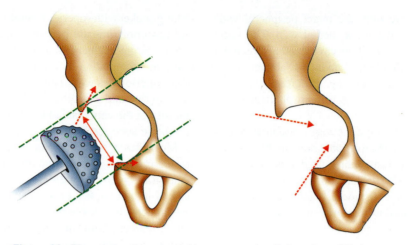

Figure 14: Divergent walls reshaped to convergent walls by using a little larger reamer than the mouth of the acetabulum

is templated for stabilization at the rim where walls start converging medially.

d. To plan the level of neck osteotomy for maintaining equal limb length.

2. Ensure availability of the bone grafts and metal reinforcements if defects are extensive.

Surgical Technique

In protrusio, the structural support for the acetabular component is provided by the peripheral walls as the inadequate and deficient floor cannot be depended upon.

A standard posterior, lateral or any other approach, one is familiar with may be used. Sciatic nerve is quite close to the hip joint in protrusio, so should be carefully protected in the posterior approach. Dislocation of the hip is often difficult because of deepened acetabulum, deformities and soft tissue contractures. Hip is mobilized by circumferential capsular release. The rim osteophytes, if any, are chiselled off. In a posterior approach gluteus maximus tendon may need to be divided partially, about 0.5-1 cm from its femoral insertion at gluteal tuberosity. This enables the proximal femur to be retracted more easily for a good acetabular exposure. Dislocation is done very gently being careful and avoiding excessive rotational maneuver as it can lead to a spiral fracture of the shaft of femur in an

osteoporotic bone. In severe protrusio, an osteotomy of the neck is often required if dislocation does not seem probable; head of the femur is extracted by a cork screw. If the mouth of the acetabulum is narrow for delivering the intact head, it may be removed in piecemeal. A low neck osteotomy may be helpful for better exposure of the acetabulum in a stiff hip.

Preparation of the acetabulum also requires a special attention because of the weak medial wall and an oblong shape of the acetabulum that may happen in supero-medial migration of the head of femur. In an oblong socket, the peripheral walls become divergent medially instead of normal convergent configuration. Also besides a medial defect there is a superior segmental deficiency as well. For stability of the implant, the divergent peripheral walls need to be reshaped to the convergent hemispherical shape. This is achieved by slightly enlarging the mouth of the socket by reaming with a little larger sized reamer than the mouth (Figure 14).

In contrast to the techniques used for normal acetabulum, in protrusio, initiation of the reaming is not started with smaller reamers due to the weak and membranous medial wall. The floor is curetted of all the soft tissues and is simply made rough and scratched by a spiked ring curette or any other instrument. Reaming of the acetabulum is started with the largest size of reamer that just fits into the mouth of the acetabulum (A-P diameter of the acetabulum).

This is to prepare only the intact peripheral walls without reaming the weak medial wall. The initial reamer should nearly fill the cavity and is directed in the anatomical direction of about 40° abduction and 20° anteversion for reaming. Progressively larger reamers are used to create a hemispherical socket peripherally.

Reaming should be done very cautiously, taking care not to destroy the available bone in the deficient acetabulum. The last reamer used shall reveal the size of the acetabulum component to be used and shall also estimate the defect and the amount of bone graft required to reinforce the deficiency. In an

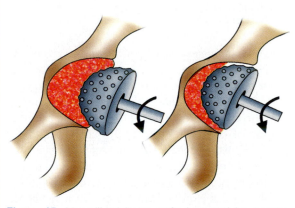

Figure 15: Morsellized bone grafts impacted by reverse reaming with a reamer 2 mm smaller than the last reamer used

oblong socket with superior migration, as the anterior and posterior rims are prepared one should not use further larger reamers to ream up to the superior dome in a temptation to seat the cup flush with host bone superiorly as well. This shall ream and eat away the anterior and posterior walls compromising the stability of the cup. Instead the superior defect if any should be bone grafted.

Morsellized cancellous bone grafts of 1-3 mm in size prepared with a bone mill or else particulate bone grafts prepared with an acetabular reamer are packed into the defect of the acetabulum. The grafts are impacted by a dome pusher or by reverse reaming with a reamer 2 mm smaller than the size of the last reamer used until sufficient thickness is achieved (Figure 15). After bone graft reconstruction, the trial cup should be at the level of the rim of the acetabulum and should have a full bony cover. Autograft bone is usually sufficient in mild to moderate protrusio because of the availability of femoral head and the acetabular reamings.

Uncemented Socket

After hemispherical preparation of the periphery of the acetabulum and bone graft reconstruction, a larger sized hemispherical porous coated acetabular component is secured and stabilized at the rim of the acetabulum in about 40° of abduction and 15-25° of anteversion (Figures 16A and B).

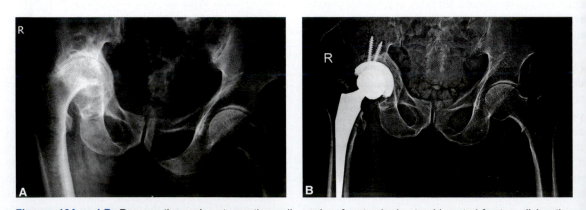

Figures 16A and B: Preoperative and postoperative radiographs of protrusio due to old central fracture dislocation reconstructed by cementless socket. Medial bone grafts and large cementless cup with a peripheral rim fixation used for reconstruction

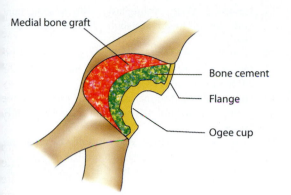

Figure 17: Flanged OGEE cemented cup – cemented over the medial bone grafts. Large superior flange helps cement pressurization and an inferior anatomical placement of the cup

Cemented Socket

The acetabulum is prepared at the periphery as usual. Multiple holes, especially in the superior dome and ischium, are drilled with 4.5 mm drill bit for a good cement fixation. Bone cement mix in the doughy state is placed directly on the grafts and pressurized with a dome pusher. The appropriate sized polyethylene cup is cemented in about 40-45° of abduction and 15-25° of anteversion. A flanged OGEE acetabular cup may be a better option since it provides a good cement pressurization and extra fixation at the rim of acetabulum. Also, because of a superior flange, a smaller OGEE cup can be used which shall provide near normal center of rotation by cementing the cup inferiorly and laterally (Figure 17).

The femoral component implantation and the rest of the procedure of arthroplasty is completed in the usual manner.

Relocation of the hip may occasionally pose some problems due to gain in length owing to acetabular reconstruction (Figures 18A and B). The following steps could be helpful:
1. Release of tight capsule, especially of inferior and anterior capsule.
2. Release/lengthening of other tight soft tissues and musculotendinous structures, i.e. ilio-psoas and fascia lata.

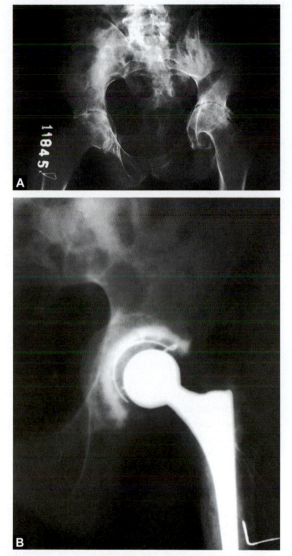

Figures 18A and B: Preoperative and postoperative radiograph of B/L protrusio following rheumatoid arthritis. Reconstruction done with a flanged cemented cup on left side

3. A larger offset stem may be used to facilitate a difficult reduction but there is a risk of greater trochanter avulsion especially in lateral approach.
4. A low neck osteotomy may be done to avoid lengthening. Here a high offset design stem may be required to avoid impingement of the greater trochanter with acetabular rim.

POSTOPERATIVE

1. Active and passive range of motion in the first 24-48 hours.
2. Non-weight bearing walking with crutch or walker for 6 weeks.
3. Partial weight bearing walking with crutch or walker up to 3 months until the bone graft appears to be incorporated on roentgenograms.
4. Full weight bearing at 3 months.

REFERENCES

1. Bayley JC, Christie MJ, Ewald FC, et al. Long-term results of total hip arthroplasty in protrusio acetabuli. J Arthroplasty 1987;2:275-9.
2. Berry DJ, Muller ME. Revision arthroplasty using an anti-protrusio cage for massive acetabular bone deficiency. J Bone Joint Surg Br 1992;74:711-5.
3. Coventry MB. The treatment of fracture dislocation of the hip by total hip arthroplasty. J Bone Joint Surg 1974;56A:1128-34.
4. Crowninshield RD, Brand RA, Pedersen DR. A stress analysis of acetabular reconstruction in protrusio acetabuli. J Bone Joint Surg 1983;65A: 495-9.
5. Garcia-Cimbrelo E, Diaz Martin A, Madero R, Munera L. Loosening of the cup after low friction Arthroplasty in patients with acetabular protrusion – The importance of the position of the cup. J Bone Joint Surg 2000;82B:108-15.
6. Gates HS, McCollum DE, Poletti SC, et al. Bone grafting in total hip arthroplasty for protrusio acetabuli. J Bone Joint Surg 1990;72A:248-51.
7. Gates HS, Poletti SC, Callaghan JJ, et al. Radiographic measurements in protrusio acetabuli. J Arthroplasty 1989;4:347-51.
8. Goodman SB, Adler SJ, Fyhrie DP, et al. The acetabular teardrop and its relevance to acetabular migration. Clin Orthop 1988;236:199.
9. Gross AE, Allan G, Catre Mel, Garbuz DS, Stockley I. Bone grafts in hip replacement surgery–The pelvic side. Orthop. Clinics of North America 1993;24:679-95.
10. Hall FM, Mauch PM, Levene MB, et al. Protrusio acetabuli following pelvic irradiation. AJR Am J Roentgenol 1979;132:291-3.
11. Harris WH. Management of the deficient acetabulum using cementless fixation without bone grafting. Orthop Clin North Am 1993;24:663-5.
12. Hastings DE, Parker SM. Protrusio acetabuli in rheumatoid arthritis. Clin Orthop 1975;108:76-83.
13. Heywood AWB. Arthroplasty with a solid bone graft for protrusio acetabuli. J Bone Joint Surg 1980;62B:332-6.
14. Hirst P, Esser M, Murphy JC, et al. Bone grafting for protrusio acetabuli during total hip replacement. J Bone Joint Surg 1987;69B:229-33.
15. Hubbard MJS. The measurement of progression in protrusio acetabuli. J Bone Joint Surg 1969;106B 506-9.
16. Jasty, Murali, Harris WH: Results of total hip reconstruction using acetabular mesh in patients with central acetabular deficiency. Clin Orthop 1988; 237 142-9.
17. Kinzinger PJ, Karthaus RP, Sloof TJ. Bone grafting for acetabular protrusion in hip arthroplasty. 27 cases of rheumatoid arthritis followed for 2-8 years. Acta Orthop Scand 1991; 62:110-12.
18. Kohler A. Roentgenology: The borderlands of the normal and the early pathological in skiagram (2nd edn). London: Balliere, Tindall and Cox, 1953.p.222
19. Kwong LM, Jasty M, Harris WH. High failure rate of bulk femoral head allografts in total hip acetabular reconstructions at 10 years. J Arthroplasty. 1993; 8:341-6.
20. McBroom RJ, Muller ME. Aseptic loosening – 15 years experience with the Muller total hip Arthroplasty. Torronto Hip Course, Feb 26, 1984.
21. McCollum DE, Nunley JA, Harrelson JM. Bone grafting in total hip replacement for acetabular protrusion. J Bone Joint Surg 1980;62A:1065-73.
22. Oh I, Harris WH. Design concepts, indications, and surgical technique for use of the protrusio shell. Clin Orthop 1982;162:175-84.
23. Overgaard K. Otto's disease and other forms of protrusio acetabuli. Acta Radiol {diag.}(Stockh.) 1935;16:390.
24. Pagnano W, Hannssen AD, Lewallen DG, et al. The effect of superior placement of the acetabular component on the rate of loosening in after total hip arthroplasty. J Bone Joint Surg 1996;78A:1004-14.
25. Ragnar J, Leif E, Stefan Z, Lars L. Total hip replacement with spongious bone graft for acetabular protrusion in patients with rheumatoid arthritis. Acta Orthop Scand 1984;55:510-13.
26. Ranawat CS, Dorr LD, Inglis AE. Total hip arthroplasty in protrusio of rheumatoid arthritis. J Bone Joint Surg 1980;62A:1059-65.
27. Ranawat CS, Zahn MG. The role of grafting in correction of protrusio acetabuli by total hip arthroplasty. J Arthroplasty 1986;1:131-7.
28. Russotti GM, Harris WH. Proximal placement of the acetabular component in total hip arthroplasty.

A long-term follow-up study. J Bone Joint Surg 1991;73:587-92.

29. Salvati EA, Bullough P, Wilson PD Jr. Intrapelvic protrusion of the acetabular component following total hip replacement. Clin Orthop 1975;111:212-27.

30. Samuel Van de Velde, Ramona Fillman and Suzzane Yandove. Protrusio acetabuli in Marfan's syndrome. History, diagnosis and treatment. J Bone Joint Surg 2006;88:639-46.

31. Schatzker J, Hastings DE, Broom RJ. Acetabular reinforcement in total hip replacement. Acta Orthop Traumat. Surg. 1979;94:135-41.

32. Schertlin: Ueber einen fall von intrapelviner varwolbung und centraler wandering der huftpfanne (Otto–Chrobaksches Becken). Beitrage sur Klinischen Chirurg. 1910;71:406-19.

33. Schreurs BW, Sloof TJJH, Buma P, et al. Acetabular reconstruction with impacted morsellized cancellous bone graft & cement. J Bone Joint Surg 1998;80-B:391-5.

34. Sloof TJJH, Huiskes R,Horn JV, Lemmens AL. Bone grafting in total hip replacement for acetabular protrusion. Acta Orthop Scand 1984;55 : 593-96.

35. Sotelo-Garza A, Charnley J. The results of Charnley arthroplasty of the hip performed for protrusio acetabuli. Clin Orthop. 1978;132:12-18.

36. Wiberg G. Shelf operation in congenital dysplasia of the acetabulum and subluxation and dislocation of the hip. J Bone Joint Surg. 1953;35A:65-80.

6 | Total Hip Replacement After Girdlestone Arthroplasty

Chandeep Singh, Albert D' Souza, SKS Marya

Excision arthroplasty is one of the oldest surgical procedures described for the treatment of pathologic conditions of the hip joint. It was initially described in the 19th century for the treatment of infected hips and then used for all kind of painful conditions around the hip. The surgery was popularized and named after the British physician G.R. Girdlestone who first reported his technique for treatment of hip tuberculosis in 1923. He advocated the resection of the femoral head and neck and a portion of the lateral aspect of the acetabulum for the treatment of advanced tuberculosis and pyogenic infections.[1-3] The indications for the original Girdlestone arthroplasty (primary) have decreased and now such extensive removal of bone and muscle mass is avoided. In today's era, the procedure of resection arthroplasty has moved from a primary procedure (for septic hips, coxarthrosis, and ankylosing spondylitis) to a salvage procedure largely for the management of infected total hip arthroplasties. It is usually a first stage procedure for management of infected total hip arthroplasty and is used as a last resort in patients with, risk of recurrent infection, poor general condition or severe loss of bone stock which may not be suited for further major interventions, especially one- or two-stage reimplantation after failed primary total hip replacement. Functional results after resection arthroplasty have been unclear ranging from poor to satisfactory with considerable pain relief and control of infection but compromising on the functional results.[4-6]

Girdlestone first reported his technique in 1928 for treatment of hip tuberculosis.[3] Fifteen years later he described the procedure in detail for treatment of hip sepsis.[7] His technique consisted of a transverse lateral approach with removal of a large wedge of the gluteus medius, minimus, and maximus including the greater trochanter. Removal of the femoral head and neck exposed the acetabulum. All acetabular cartilage and the superior rim of the acetabulum were removed. Occasionally a medial approach, excising a wedge of the adductors and pectineus and sparing the neurovascular structures, was used. There have been instances where an additional medial incision has been described. Conversion of a classical Girdlestone arthroplasty to a total hip replacement would be very difficult, in view of the absence of the abductor musculature and with the likely presence of acetabular deficiency.[7] Fortunately the majority of hip excision arthroplasties that a surgeon is likely to see in his current practice would not have undergone such an extensive resection. Recent authors have advocated the importance of maximal preservation of proximal femoral bone stock and making every effort to preserve the abductor musculature. Grauer et al[8] described four possible levels of proximal femoral resection: Type I—a substantial portion of the femoral neck remains, usually performed for failed resurfacings, Type II—a small portion of the femoral neck remains, Type III—intertrochanteric resection, Type IV—subtrochanteric resection. The obvious clinical implication of this classification is that the more proximal the resection, the better is the overall function, walking and activity of the patient. However, the correlation between the clinical result and the radiological classification has been found to be lacking by a few studies. But the implication on the conversion to a total hip can be clearly correlated with the availability of a better bone stock.[5,9]

In recent times Girdlestone excision arthroplasty is used for treatment of infected total hip arthroplasty. Two stage revisions is the norm nowadays with an intervening period of resection of all components and removal of cement followed by reimplantation. The decision to perform a resection arthroplasty without reimplantation of a second prosthesis is based upon multiple factors. Important considerations include infection with multiple organisms or bacteria resistant to antibiotic therapy, poor quality local soft tissues, unacceptable complexity of the reconstruction, refusal by the patient to have another operation after removal of the implant, and patients with systemic disease, poor overall health, inadequate bone stock or combinations of these factors.[10-17]

Patient satisfaction after Girdlestone has been reviewed by various authors, a high mortality and a poor functional outcome could be attributed to a higher age group, poor general health and highly selected group of patients, who were unfit for reimplantation surgery. In case it is done in younger age group or a more mobile patient's the level of dissatisfaction has been seen.[4,6,18]

Nonetheless, the conversion of a Girdlestone arthroplasty to a total hip replacement has been described as "one of the greatest challenges in adult reconstructive surgery".[19] These procedures demand comprehensive preoperative clinical evaluation as well as detailed laboratory and radiological investigations. The availability of appropriate armamentarium of instruments and implants has to be ensured before undertaking this procedure.

These are a few points to be taken into consideration before undertaking the conversion form Girdlestone arthroplasty to total hip. There are a lot of reasons for the dissatisfaction of patients and we would just like to discuss a few of them so that the evaluation is done preoperatively and the expected difficulties are better understood.

Gait after Girdlestone excision arthroplasty has been mentioned as ungainly and difficult requiring a lot of energy. The use of walking support has been documented by Walters et al[20] wherein of the nine patients only one could walk without any support. Clinical examination of the patients with excision arthroplasty reveals a positive Trendelenburg test with an abductor lurch while walking. McElwaine et al.[21] and Clegg[22] reviewed patients with excision arthroplasty after infected prosthesis removal and found that majority of them walked poorly as compared to the gait before hip replacement.

Substantial limb length inequality has been seen in all excision arthroplasty which in turn is responsible for the instability and gait difficulties. Shortening may range for 3 to 11 cm but most commonly is around 4 to 6 cm.[16,23] Postoperative traction or ischial weight bearing caliper has no bearing on final shortening but it does correlate with the level of femoral neck resection. The limb length discrepancy is usually addressed with shoe raise, which itself may be a reason for the younger patient to ask for restoration of the limb length by replacement.

Preoperative Evaluation

The purpose of the evaluation is to ensure that the conversion procedure is appropriate to the general condition of the patient, to rule out any ongoing infective process and to assess the available bony and soft deficiency (Figure 1). As in every clinical condition a detailed history of the patient is a must which should also document the reasons as to why be the patient asking for a conversion now.

Original Records

If the procedure was performed elsewhere, every effort should be made to get a copy of the operation notes and the hospital medical records. These should be scanned for the reasons why the surgery was performed, the presurgery functional status, the culture reports at that time and also the condition of the bones and the abductor musculature at that time.

Physical Examination

This should include both a general physical examination and an detailed local examination of the hip. The general examination should assess any remote source of infection, spine examination and the upper limb strength to support the use of walking aid if required. Attention should be paid to any previous incisions, healed sinus tracts, true and apparent shortening, the presence of palpable abductor activity and movement at the pseudoarthrosis.

Neurovascular examination and documentation is a must before undertaking this venture.

Labs

Useful blood investigations include inflammatory markers like ESR and C-reactive protein (CRP). The white blood cell count is rarely elevated in chronic hip infections and in general not useful in guiding treatment. ESR and CRP have been guiding orthopedic surgeons for long but more recently they have been found to be less accurate as they are also influenced by the hosts inflammatory conditions. Spangehl et al.[24] have found that a combination should be used and they found it to be more useful. Elevated levels of the cytokine interleukin-6 (IL-6), a factor that is produced by monocytes and macrophages, have recently been shown to be correlated positively with the presence of chronic periprosthetic infection. With a normal serum IL-6, defined as 10 pg/ml, the test has a sensitivity, specificity, positive predictive value, negative predictive value, and accuracy of 100%, 95%, 89%, 100% and 97%.[13] Unfortunately, the levels of IL-6 may be elevated in patients with chronic inflammatory disease such as rheumatoid arthritis.[25]

Aspiration

Aspiration should be routinely undertaken if the initial procedure was done for infective reasons. It is imperative that the patient should not take antibiotics for at least 4 weeks prior to the aspiration. The aspiration should preferable be done under image intensifier maintain asepsis at all times. The aspiration of a pseudoarthrosis presents certain technical difficulties. The acetabulum and the femoral shaft may be filled with fibrous tissue and the localization of the fluid might pose difficulty.[26] If no fluid is obtainable then the use of core biopsy needles may be considered and the tissues sent for culture. Polymerase chain reaction (PCR) techniques have been investigated in the quest to detect subclinical joint infections. The ability to amplify minute levels of bacterial DNA to detectable levels should in theory improve our diagnostic accuracy of periprosthetic infections. However present techniques are insensitive due to problems of contamination and result in a high rate of false positives.[27] With further refinement these techniques may be applicable in the future.

Radiography

The aim is to clearly define the available bone stock and to measure the limb length discrepancy. Initial evaluation is should be with plain radiography, an anteroposterior view of the pelvis and a full length AP and lateral view of the femur is desired. A CT scan of the pelvis at times is helpful in assessing the bone loss at the acetabulum which can prepare us better with planning for the implants needed (Figures 1 and 2).

Timing of Revision Surgery

The ideal length of interval between stages has not been determined but by convention waiting for minimum of 6 weeks is recommended. Ketterl et al[28] found that reimplantation carried out as early as 4 weeks (average 2.1 weeks) was better than reimplantation at 44 weeks (average 12.7 weeks), with respect to function, mortality and cure of infection. At our center after the first-stage procedure, an organism-specific intravenous (IV) antibiotic regimen is recommended if there is no growth the antibiotic should be started in consultation with the microbiologist for a minimum of 6 weeks. The IV antibiotics are stopped when the acute phase reactants have returned to normal, and a 2-week period without antibiotics then ensues. The patient is followed clinically for any evidence of re-emergence of the infection. Aspiration is performed to confirm the absence of infection. Factors that will delay implantation include a persistently elevated ESR level, recurrent local infection or positive repeat aspiration culture. Reimplantation may not be appropriate in patients with poor general health, dementia, a history of substance abuse or in an immunocompromised patients.

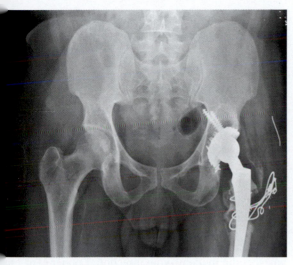

Figure 1: Preoperative infected THR

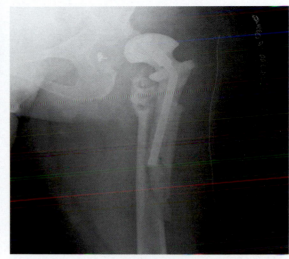

Figure 2: Postoperative with Prostalac spacer

In case of traditional Girdlestone arthroplasty Rittmeister et al.[29] had hypothesized that patients with a shorter duration of Girdlestone arthroplasty would do better compared to those with a longer duration. However, their findings did not support this contention. In a study of 16 patients with conversion arthroplasty, Schroeder et al.[18] suggested that 12 months would be the optimal interval between removal and conversion, however it remains unclear on what basis this conclusion is drawn.

Surgical Approach

A few points to be kept in mind before undertaking the reconstruction:
- The femur is typically medialized and may be fixed in adduction, resulting in a narrow soft tissue sleeve between the femur and the pelvis.
- Proximal migration of the femoral shaft is always present requiring substantial lengthening. This would require extensive mobilization of the proximal femur and at times exposure of the sciatic nerve.
- Comprehensive exposure of the acetabulum is a must to permit its identification and also to quantify and reconstruct the acetabular defects.
- The reconstruction of femur might require use of strut or allografts and at times correction of angular deformities if present.

- Abductor musculatures condition is highly variable. They may be intact or excised or interposed between the femur and the acetabulum. The continuity of the greater trochanter needs to be assessed both pre- and intraoperatively.

The choice of the surgical approach is usually the surgeons. Rittmeister et al.[29] and Dallari et al.[30] have preferred the anterolateral approach for the procedure. Eric M et al.[31] have described the use of the posterior approach. In hip surgery as we all are aware presence of scars does not determine the use of the approach. If any adherent scars are present then a plastic surgery consult should be considered. The advantage of the posterior approach lies in the exposure of the sciatic nerve and the assessment on table of the stretch on it.

The use of the trochanteric slide osteotomy has been described to expose the proximal femur. If no trochanter is present then the soft tissue envelope consisting of the gluteal abductors and vasti in continuity is elevated as described by Mcfarland and Osborne.[32] A vastus slide approach has also being mentioned as a modification of the above approach.[33]

Presence of Cement Beads or Spacers

Acrylic bone cement is a very effective local delivery system for heat-stable antibiotics, and concentrations

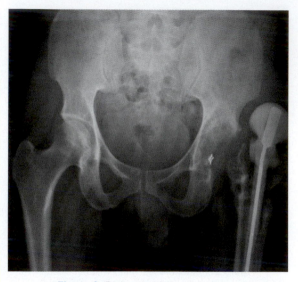

Figure 3: Dislocated Prostalac spacer

have been measured in resected joint spaces that exceed the systemic levels (Figure 3). The utility of the cement–antibiotic composite for infected implants was first described by Buchholz and coworkers[34] in 1970 for prophylaxis and one-stage exchange. The antibiotic-loaded cement spacer concept was later introduced initially in the form of beads[35] and has since been described in many other configurations. Current literature clearly demonstrates that the use of antibiotic-impregnated cement in any configuration improves the results. Cement beads, other non-articulating forms, and monopolar endoprosthetic designs have all been utilized over a period of time.

The removal of cement beads requires patience and accurate identification. The chains should be removed by gentle traction in the line in which they were inserted combined with careful dissection of the intervening soft tissues. Disastrous complications both vascular and neural have been reported in removal of these chains. However with increased availability of endoprosthetic design spacers the use of beads around the hip has gone down. The concept of the spacers has advantages over beads, in that it maintains leg length and tissue tension, can be used when there are major bone deficits, and allows enough stability for mobilization of the patient. Various authors have mentioned reimplantation of

the final prosthetic is significantly easier after the use of such a device, and the functional capacity of the patient is improved much earlier.[36,37]

Intraoperative Specimens

Unlike a primary hip arthroplasty it is wiser to withhold the preoperative antibiotics and the antibiotics is to be given only after obtaining samples for culture and frozen section. It is wise to obtain three samples for culture as it more likely to rule out contamination. Intraoperative Gram stains of joint fluid and tissue have proven unreliable and are no longer factored into the decision-making process.[38]

Frozen section has been reported as both sensitive and specific in identifying infection. Lonner et al[39] in a prospective study on 175 revision total joint arthroplasties (142 hip and 33 knee), reported a sensitivity of 84%, specificity of 96%, positive predictive value of 70% and negative predictive value of 98% in identifying infections when a positive result was defined as at least five polymorphonuclear cells per high power-field at microscopy. When an index of at least 10 polymorphonuclear cells per high-power field was used the sensitivity and negative predictive value remained the same but the specificity increased to 99% and the positive predictive value increased significantly to 89%.

Factors in Achieving Limb Length

A number of factors need to be considered in any attempt to restore limb length during conversion of resection arthroplasty to a total hip replacement. These include methods of mobilizing proximal femur, identification of the true acetabulum, preservation of a functional abductor mechanism and avoidance of sciatic nerve injury.

Following the initial exposure the proximal femur must be released from the dense scar tissue surrounding it in the upper end. It may involve delivering the proximal femur out of the wound and gently clearing the upper end with help of a cautery or scalpel. Particular attention needs to be paid to the medial tissue and iliopsoas tendon needs release most of the times. The iliopsoas tendon itself is found to be shortened and contributing to the shortening and the fixed flexion of the proximal femur.

When the femur has been mobilized it should be retracted anteriorly or posteriorly and the acetabulum needs to be identified. Working carefully the fibrous tissue is removed and an attempt is made to work distally and put the inferior retractor in the obturator foramen or the cotyloid notch of the ischium, thus defining the inferior margin of the true acetabulum. The failure to identify the true acetabulum can result in high cup placement.

The management of the abductors is the key, on one hand a trochanteric osteotomy helps in the surgical exposure, while on the other stable fixation and reduction of the trochanter after substantial lengthening may be difficult to achieve and may predispose to instability and failure of fixation devices. An attempt should be made to maintain the functional continuity by preserving the aponeurosis over the greater trochanter. It is also suggested to accept a slight fixed abduction at the hip.

Cementless vs Cemented Implants

The advantage of using cement lies in the ability to add antibiotic, which elutes over time, keeping infection in check. Indeed, early successful reimplantations involved use of antibiotic laden cemented prostheses. Buccholz et al.[34] introduced the concept of antibiotic impregnated cement and popularized its use in Europe for single stage revision surgery, reporting infection cure rates of 77% in his series. Raut et al.[40] reported a success rate of 84% using the same treatment strategy. A review of published series comparing use of plain bone cement and antibiotic impregnated cement in single-stage revisions found cumulative success rates of 60% and 83%, respectively, strongly suggesting there was no role for single-stage cementless revisions.[41]

The superiority of cementless hip revisions over cemented implants in aseptic loosening led investigators to consider their use in two-stage reimplantations (Figures 4A and B). The limited time dependant ability of antibiotic to elute from bone cement in sufficient quantities to overcome infective bacteria coupled with the negative long-term effects of cement on the function of polymorphonuclear cells supported the move towards cementless two-stage reimplantations. Fehring et al.[42] demonstrated a success rate of 92% (25 patients) at average 41 months follow-up using a two-stage cementless reimplantation approach. The authors highlighted the importance of using implants of appropriate design to ensure bone ingrowth of the femoral component. They used proximally milled cementless implants in cases where proximal femoral bone stock was adequate and extensively coated stems to obtain diaphyseal stability where there was proximal structural bone loss. Other authors have reported similar experience: Haddad et al.[43] (50 patients)

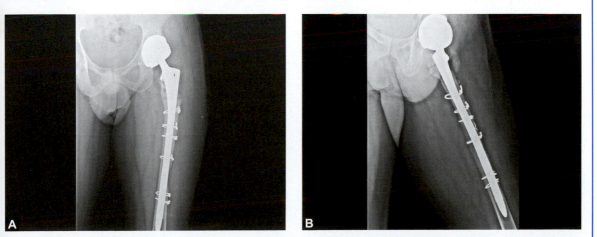

Figures 4A and B: Postoperative of the same patient with uncemented hip replacement (Extensively coated stem)

reported a 92% success rate at 5.8 years follow-up; Kraay et al.[44] (33 patients) reported a 93% success rate. Reported success rates for two- stage cemented reimplantations range from 90 to 95%.

Acetabular Cups

The acetabular bone stock is assessed and classified according to Paprosky's classification.[45] Cemented cups were used by earlier authors, keeping in mind the local antibiotic delivery advantage of cement in mind. However currently, many surgeons would recommend a two stage revision to eradicate the infection because it allows for more options for the final reconstruction and has a higher success rate for the eradication of infection. The use of cement at the second stage allows local antibiotic delivery, but the intermediate and long-term results of cemented components in the revision setting have been poor.[43,44] As a result, many surgeons prefer uncemented components for revision total hip arthroplasty.

The use of cemented cups with impaction grafting has also been used.[30] The availability of tantalum Trabecular Metal acetabular component with Trabecular Metal buttress augments has shown promising early results.[46] The trend has been to move towards uncemented implants for the revision settings.

Femoral Stem

Revision arthroplasty using cemented implants, although still widely used, is not without its detractors. The proximal femoral cancellous bed available for cement interdigitation often is deficient in a revision setting. The canal of the proximal femur often is sclerotic and smooth as a result of bone resorption and relative movement between bone and the loosened implant. As a result, the initial stability of the revised cemented prosthesis is much lower than that of the primary cemented prosthesis. The long-term results of revision total hips using cemented femoral stems, have remained unpredictable and discouraging even with impaction grafting and third generation cementing technique.[47,48]

The poor results with cemented revisions have led investigators to explore cementless options. Proximally porous-coated implants have been used extensively for revision of the failed femoral component. The proximally porous-coated implants rely on maximum bone contact in the metaphyseal region to obtain stability and eventual bone ingrowth. Unfortunately, in revision hip surgery, the environment for proximal bone ingrowth is usually not favorable because the proximal femoral bone stock is often deficient, weak, poorly vascularized, and sclerotic.

Then efforts were directed to obtain intimate diaphyseal fit and fill and biologic fixation. These efforts have led to the development of the fully coated, monoblock, cementless femoral stems. These implants relies on the diaphyseal fit and stability in the relatively normal distal femoral bone and offers less demands from the damaged proximal metaphyseal bone in the femoral revision. This technique permits reliable biologic fixation at intermediate-term and long-term follow-up.[49] The main disadvantage of those stems is related to its one piece nature; the surgeon must take critical decisions about version, offset, limb length and soft tissue balancing at once, resulting in high rate of intraoperative complications.

These problems led to the evolution of modular cementless femoral stems. Modularity in cementless femoral revision permits independent fitting of the diaphysis and metaphysis; correct adjustment of length, offset, and version to facilitate the reconstruction of the proximal femur and to offer ultimate clinical performance.

The use allograft is needed many a times; impaction grafting has been recommended by many surgeons and does give good results in expert hands. Use of structural graft with implant combination has been described by a few people, but the widespread use is limited due to lack of availability of graft.

Subtrochanteric osteotomy has been used by a few authors to get the hip center at the correct level and avoid straining the sciatic nerve. Use of S Rom stem has been recommended.[50] There have been occasional case reports of Ilizarov distraction before revision hip replacement in severe shortening following resection arthroplasty.[51]

Postoperative Management

Postoperative management is determined largely by the extent and nature of the reconstruction and will therefore; need to be individualized for each case. Some specific points which need to observed:

- Intravenous antibiotics need to be continued minimum five days, if the intraoperative cultures come sterile. In case cultures are positive then the appropriate antibiotics need to be continued for six weeks with careful observation of the patient.
- Partial sciatic nerve injuries usually recover, while the prognosis of a full sciatic nerve palsy is poor. Little is gained by re-exploration if no misplaced screw or wire can be held accountable for the same.
- The abductor mechanism might need the use of an abduction brace in the postoperative period to allow for trochanteric healing or to prevent early dislocation.
- The range of motion is less than that achieved by a primary arthroplasty and both the patient and the surgeon need to be aware of it.
- Limb length discrepancy should be only addressed once the patient has been comfortably mobilized.

Review of Literature

Literature on total hip conversion of Girdlestone arthroplasty is sparse and almost uniformly relates to the various difficulties faced in reconstruction. However if you look at the functional results they have been encouraging in majority of these few papers.

Rittmeister et al.[29] reported greater patient satisfaction and better function if Girdlestone hips were converted to a hip arthroplasty rather than being left with the excisional procedure. The incidence of postoperative complications and revisions were similar for both groups. Charlton et al.[52] in retrospective study showed a high rate of dislocation (11.4%) and persistent limp (39%) following delayed conversion. A high dislocation rate following conversion of the Girdlestone procedure to secondary total hip arthroplasty relates to soft tissue contracture, limb length discrepancy, deficient bone stock and malpositioning of the components. A constrained acetabular component should be considered to reduce the dislocation rate. Schroder et al.[53] followed two groups of patients: thirty-two patients had a long-standing pseudarthrosis; in the other group of sixteen patients, a total hip replacement was reimplanted at an average of 3 years after a pseudarthrosis. The improvement in hip function after the reimplantation was marginal and the results were comparable to a well-functioning pseudarthrosis. Personal satisfaction and the activities of daily living were marginally better in the reimplantation group, (Harris hip score 64 compared to 58 in those with a pseudarthrosis). Brandt et al.[54] stated that prosthesis removal and delayed reimplantation arthroplasty is an effective treatment to limit the recurrence of *Staphylococcus aureus* prosthetic joint infection, provided there is no evidence of infection at the time of reimplantation arthroplasty. Dante Dallari et al.[31] performed a retrospective review of 16 patients and mention a significant reduction in limb length discrepancy and an improvement in the walking ability. They have favored doing this procedure for younger patients (<65 years).

CONCLUSION

Conversion of Girdlestone excision arthroplasty to total hip replacement is usually technically feasible given the advances made in the implants; however it requires careful preoperative planning, patient selection and considerable experience in reconstruction techniques. Major intraoperative considerations include restoration of length, avoidance of sciatic nerve injury and maintaining the abductor mechanism. Identifying and managing the residual sepsis prior to the revision surgery is paramount. Careful preoperative planning should be done to identify the bone deficiency so that necessary tools and techniques are available in the operating room.

REFERENCES

1. Girdlestone GR. Acute pyogenic arthritis of the hip. Clin Orthop 1982;170:3-7.
2. Girdlestone GR. Acute pyogenic arthritis of the hip. Lancet 1943;1:419-421.
3. Girdlestone GR. Arthrodesis and other operations for tuberculosis of the hip. In: The Robert Jones Birthday Volume. A Collection of Surgical Essays. London: Oxford University Press; 1928:347.
4. Grauer JD, Amstutz HC, O'Carroll PF, et al. Resection arthroplasty of the hip. J Bone Joint Surg 1989;71A:669-678.
5. Ballard WT, Lowery DA, Brand RA. Resection arthroplasty of the hip. J Arthroplasty 1995;10:772-779.
6. Scott JC. Pseudoarthrosis of the hip. Clin Orthop 1963;31:31-38.
7. Hanssen AD, Mariani EM, Kavanagh BF, Coventry MB. Resection arthroplasty (Girdlestone procedure) nerve palsies, limb length inequality and osteolysis following total hip arthroplasty. In: Morrey BF ed. Joint replacement arthroplasty. New York: Churchill Livingstone 1991;891-905.
8. Grauer JD, Amstutz HC, O'Carroll PF, et al. Resection arthroplasty of the hip. J Bone Joint Surg 1989;71A:669-678.
9. Haw CS, Gray DH. Excision arthroplasty of the hip. J Bone Joint Surg Br 1976;58:44-7.
10. Garvin KL, Fitzgerald RH Jr, Salvati EA, et al. Reconstruction of the infected total hip and knee arthroplasty with gentamicin-impregnated Palacos bone cement. Instr Course Lect 1993;42:293-302.
11. Mont MA, Waldman BJ, Hungerford DS. Evaluation of preoperative cultures before second-stage reimplantation of a total knee prosthesis complicated by infection: a comparison-group study. J Bone Joint Surg [Am] 2000;82-A:1552-7.
12. Springer BD, Lee GC, Osmon D, et al. Systemic safety of high-dose antibiotic loaded cement spacers after resection of an infected total knee arthroplasty. Clin Orthop 2004;427:47-51.
13. Lieberman JR, Callaway GH, Salvati EA, Pellicci PM, Brause BD. Treatment of the infected total hip arthroplasty with a two-stage reimplantation protocol. Clin Orthop 1994;301:205-12.
14. Colyer RA, Capello WN. Surgical treatment of the infected hip implant: two-stage reimplantation with a one-month interval. Clin Orthop 1994;298:75-9.
15. Garvin KL, Evans BG, Salvati EA, Brause BD. Palacos gentamicin for the treatment of deep periprosthetic hip infections. Clin Orthop 1994;298:97-105.
16. Bourne RB, Hunter GA, Rorabeck CH, Macnab JJ. A six-year follow-up of infected total hip replacements managed by Girdlestone's arthroplasty. J Bone Joint Surg Br 1984;66:340-3.
17. Muller R, Schlegel KF, Konermann H. Long-term results of the Girdlestone hip. Arch Orthop Trauma Surg 1989;108:359-62.
18. Schröder J, Saris D, Besselaar PP, Marti RK. Comparison of the results of the Girdlestone pseudarthrosis with reimplantation of a total hip replacement. Int Orthop 1998;22:215-8.
19. Berman AT, Mazur T. Conversion of resection arthroplasty to total hip replacement. Orthopedics 1994;17:1155-8.
20. Walters RL, Perry J, Contay P, Lunsforb O'Mearap. The energy cost of walking with arthritis of the hip and knee. Clin orthop 1987;214:278-284
21. McElwaine JP, Colville J. Excision arthroplasty for infected total hip replacements. J Bone Joint Surg Br 1984;66:168-71.
22. Clegg J. The results of the pseudarthrosis after removal of an infected total hip prosthesis. J Bone Joint Surg Br 1977;59:298–301.
23. Ahlgren SA, Gudmundsson G, Bartholdsson E. Function after removal of a septic total hip prosthesis. A survey of 27 Girdlestone hips. Acta Orthop Scand 1980;51:541-5.
24. Spangehl MJ, Masri BA, O'Connell JX, Duncan CP. Prospective analysis of preoperative and intraoperative investigations for the diagnosis of infection at the sites of two hundred and two revision total hip arthroplasties. J Bone Joint Surg [Am] 1999;81:672-83.
25. Fitzgerald RH. Infected total hip arthroplasty: diagnosis and treatment. J Am Acad Orthop Surg 1995;3:249-62.
26. Swan JS, braustein EM, capello W. Aspiration of the hip inpatients treated with Girdlestone arthroplasty. Am J Radiol 1991;156:454-546.
27. Clarke MT, Roberts CP, Lee PTH, Gray J, Keene GS, Rushton N. Polymerase chain reaction can detect bacterial DNA in aseptical loose total hip arthroplasties. Clin Orthop 2004;427:132-7.
28. Ketterl R, Henly MB, Strubinger B, et al. Analysis of three operative techniques for infected total hip replacements. Orthop Trans 1998;12:715.

29. Rittmeister M, Manthei L, Muller M, Hailer NP. Reimplantation of the artificial hip joint in Girdlestone hips is superior to Girdlestone arthroplasty by itself. Z Orthop Ihre Grenzgeb 2004;142:559-63.

30. Dante Dallari, Milena Fini, Chiara Carubbi O, Gianluca Giavaresi, Nicola Rani Nicolandrea Del Piccolo, Maria Sartori, Alessandra Maso. Total hip arthroplasty after excision arthroplasty:indications and limits. Hip Int 2011;21(04):436-40.

31. Eric masterson, Bassam A. Masri Clive P. Conversion of Girdlestone arthroplasty to total hip replacement. In: James V Bono (ed): Revision Total Hip Replacement. Springer 505-516.

32. Mcfarland B, OsborneG. Approach to the hup: a suggested improvement on kochers method. J Bone Joint surg Br 1954;36:354.

33. Glassman AH, Engh CA, Bobyn JD. A technique of extensile exposure for total hip arthroplasty. J Arthroplasty 1987;36:364-67.

34. Buchholz HW, Elson RA, Engelbrecht E, et al. Management of deep infection in total hip replacement. J Bone Joint Surg 1981;63(B)342-353.

35. Hovelius L, Josefsson G. An alternative method for exchange operation of infected arthroplasty. Acta Orthop Scand 1979;50:93-6.

36. Duncan CP, Beauchamp C. A temporary antibiotic-loaded joint replacement system for management of complex infections involving the hip. Orthop Clin North Am 1993;24:751-59.

37. Masri B, Duncan CP, Beauchamp CP. Long-term elution of antibiotics from bone cement: An *in vivo* study suing the PROSTALAC system. J Arthroplasty 1998;13:331-338.

38. Della Valle CJ, Zuckerman JD, Di Cesare PE. Periprosthetic sepsis. Clin Orthop 2004;420:26-31.

39. Lonner JH, Desai P, Di Cesare PE, Steiner G, Zuckerman JD. The reliability of analysis on intraoperative frozen sections for identifying active infection during revision hip or knee arthroplasty. J Bone Joint Surg [Am] 1996;78:1553-8.

40. Raut VV, Siney PD, Wroblewski BM. One-stage revision of total hip arthroplasty for deep infection. Long-term followup. Clin Orthop 1995;321:202-7.

41. Hanssen AD, Rand JA. Evaluation and treatment of infection at the site of a total hip or knee arthroplasty. Instruct Course Lecture 1999;48:111-22.

42. Fehring TK, Calton TF, Griffin WL. Cementless fixation in two-stage reimplantation for periprosthetic sepsis. J Anthroplasty 1999;14(2):175-81.

43. Haddad FS, Muirhead-Allwood SK, Manktelow ARJ, Bacarese-Hamilton I. Two-stage uncemented revision hip arthroplasty for infection. J Bone Joint Surg [Br] 2000;82-(B):689-94.

44. Kraay MJ, Goldberg VM, Fitzgerald SJ, Salata MJ. Cementless two-staged total hip arthroplasty for deep periprosthetic infection. Clin Orthop 2005;441: 243-9.

45. Paprosky WG, Perona PG, Lawrence JM. Acetabular defect classification and surgical reconstruction in revision arthroplasty: A 6-year follow-up evaluation. J Arthroplasty 1994;9:33-44.

46. Siegmeth A, Duncan CP, Masri BA, Kim WY, Garbuz DS. Modular tantalum augments for acetabular defects in revision hip arthroplasty. Clin Orthop Relat Res 2009;467(1):199-205.

47. Mulroy WF, Estok DM, Harris WH. Revision total hip arthroplasty with use of so called second generation cementing techniques for aseptic loosening of the femoral component. J Bone Joint Surg 1996; 78(A):982.

48. Masterton EL, Masri BA, Duncan CP. The cement mantle in the Exeter impaction grafting technique. A cause for concern. J Arthroplasty 1997;12:759.

49. Mulroy WF, Estok DM, Harris WH. Revision total hip arthroplasty with use of so called second generation cementing techniques for aseptic loosening of the femoral component. J Bone Joint Surg 1996;78(A):982.

50. S. Kessler. Extensive subtrochanteric shortening osteotomy enables the conversion of a long lasting resection arthroplasty to a total hip replacement. Acta chirurgiae orthopaedicae et traumatologiae čechosl, 2008;75:306-307.

51. Mark R Brinker, Y Vasilios Mathews, Daniel P O'Connor, Y Ilizarov. Distraction before revision hip arthroplasty after resection arthroplasty with profound limb shortening. The Journal of Arthroplasty 2009;24(5).

52. Charlton WP, Hozack WJ, Teloken MA, Rao R, Bissett GA. Complications associated with reimplantation after Girdlestone arthroplasty. Clin Orthop 2003;407:119-26.

53. Schroder J, Saris D, Besselaar PP, Marti RK. Comparison of the results of the Girdlestone pseudarthrosis with reimplantation of a total hip replacement. Int Orthop 1998;22:215-8.

54. Brandt CM, Duffy MC, Berbari EF, Hanssen AD, Steckelberg JM, Osmon DR. *Staphylococcus aureus* prosthetic joint infection treated with prosthesis removal and delayed reimplantation arthroplasty. Mayo Clin Proc 1999;74:553-8.

7 | Osteoporotic Femoral Neck Fractures

Rastogi S, Shitij Kacker, SKS Marya

A hip fracture, especially a displaced femoral neck fracture, is probably the most devastating consequence of osteoporosis in the increasing elderly population and a major challenge for health care and society. Approximately 250,000 hip fractures occur in the United States alone, with 87% of these occurring in people older than 65 years and 75% of them are women.[1] By the year 2040, it is anticipated that this number of annual hip fractures will exceed 500,000. By the year 2050, 6.3 million annual hip fractures are expected to occur worldwide of which 1 million are expected to be in India.[2] Femoral neck fractures constitute approximately 50% of all hip fractures and 70-75% of these neck fractures are displaced (Garden III and IV).[3] Femoral neck fractures with osteoporosis pose a formidable challenge to the orthopedic surgeon. The population of elderly patients with femoral neck fractures comprises several subpopulations, ranging from the lucid, relatively healthy, active and independently living patient with a long-life expectancy to the institutionalized, cognitively impaired and bedridden patient with a substantially shorter life expectancy. It is universally agreed that surgical intervention leads to better results but deciding on the operative modality can be difficult. There are several treatment modalities available, i.e. internal fixation (IF), hemiarthroplasty (HA, unipolar or bipolar) and total hip replacement (THR), with each treatment modality having its unique characteristics, advantages and disadvantages (Figure 1).

Osteoporosis which is usually undiagnosed[4] is the most important risk factor for a hip fracture and consequently, most of the patients are women, approximately 70%.[1] Even after modern treatment, the individual patient has an increased mortality risk and is likely to experience a major negative impact on hip function and quality of life, which in turn may lead to a loss of autonomy. Because treatment is fraught with difficulties, fracture prevention is of paramount importance. All postmenopausal women and elderly population should undergo regular risk assessment and durel energy X-ray absorptiometry (DEXA) scanning. Patients should also receive calcium and antiresorptive therapy.

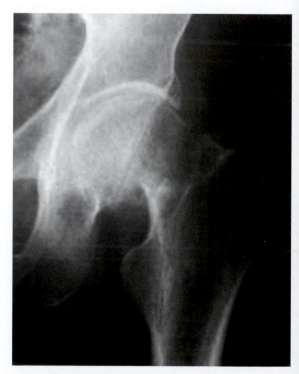

Figure 1: Fracture neck of femor displaced

ETIOLOGY

Femoral neck fractures usually occur after falls. Factors that increase the risk of these injuries are related to situations that increase the probability of falls and those that decrease the intrinsic ability of the patient to withstand trauma. The likelihood of a fall is increased with physical deconditioning, malnutrition, osteoporosis, impaired vision and difficulties with balance, dementia, neurological problems and slow reflexes.

Hence, these fractures are more common in the geriatric age group with a large number of patients having associated comorbid conditions, balance problems and dementia. Osteoporosis is one of the most important risk factors in this age group and decreases the ability of the bone to withstand trauma.

Mortality within the first year of sustaining a femoral neck fracture ranges from 20-30%.[5] The primary complications after femoral neck fractures are nonunion and avascular necrosis. The rates of these complications are varied in the literature and are dependent on number of factors including age of the patient, concomitant osteoporosis, comorbid conditions and the primary treatment received.

The epidemiological correlation between osteoporosis and femoral neck fractures is significant and well documented. Approximately 7% of all females aged 35-40 and 33% over 65 years of age suffer from osteoporosis. Nearly 40% of females aged above 50 years are at a risk of at least one osteoporotic fracture in their lifetime, the most common of which is a femoral neck fracture.[5]

The frequency of these fractures is constantly increasing due to increasing percentage of geriatric population. In 1990, 1.7 million patient's worldwide suffered hip fractures and the majority were above 50 years of age.[6] The incidence of these fractures increases dramatically after the age of 70 years.[5]

SEX

Incidences of femoral neck fractures are higher in females than males. The incidence in white females is 1 in 6.[5]

Because bone loss is greater in females than in males and with the added risk of osteoporosis following menopause, the frequency of these fractures increases exponentially with age, particularly after the age of 70 years. The cumulative risk for hip fracture is about 20% for an 80-year-old female and almost 50% for 90-year-old women.[6]

The risk of death in women with hip fractures is approximately 2-4 times greater in the first year than women without hip fracture. In females and males, the rate of femoral fracture is 17.5% and 6% respectively.[5] This is much higher than incidences of vertebral and wrist fractures. The life expectancy of a female with femoral neck fracture is reduced by 12-15%.[5] However, many studies have shown that the mortality after femoral neck fracture is higher in males than females. Men constitute approximately 33% of the annual hip fracture patients and about 1/3 of them die in the first year of injury.[5]

Race

The highest rates of hip fractures are found in white females followed by white males and the lowest incidences are in black males. It is postulated that difference in bone density of these races are responsible for this variation. Thus people of African descent have lower fracture rates than white population and Hispanic women have half as many fractures as white females despite similar peak bone mass.[5]

Osteoporosis

Senile osteoporosis usually occurs after 70 years of age and is found in both males and females. Age related bone loss starts between 35 and 40 years of age and is associated with a steady 1-2% loss of cortical and trabecular bone every year. Typically osteoporotic fractures affect the vertebral body, distal radius and proximal femur. Femoral neck fracture is a major complication of osteoporosis. Femoral neck fractures constitute about 50% of all hip fractures and 70-75% of these are displaced.[3] About 20-30% of patients who have a femoral neck fracture die within the first year of injury.[5] Half of the survivors remain disabled to some degree for life with inability to return to pre-injury activities or a pain free hip. Osteoporotic femoral neck fractures cause considerable social and economic loss and are associated with significant morbidity.

rCHAPTER 7 | 55

OSTEOPOROTIC FEMORAL NECK FRACTURES

PROTEIN ENERGY MALNUTRITION

Protein energy malnutrition (PEM) has been found in 30-50% of hip fracture patients. The combination of PEM related factors such as muscle atrophy, lack of subcutaneous fat and osteoporosis makes the elderly more prone to falls.[7] The cushioning capacity of the subcutaneous tissue diminishes[8] and the osteoporotic skeleton fractures more easily. Poor nutritional status complicates rehabilitation after a fracture[9] and postoperative rehabilitation is facilitated by actively improving nutritional intake.

Classification of Hip Fractures; Is it a Helpful Guide in Decision Making?

Classification system should provide a basis for clinical decision making and correlate with outcome. Any classification system should furthermore have a high inter and intraobserver reliability and facilitate comparison of treatment modalities between centers. Traditionally used classification system for femoral neck fractures includes Gardens classification, Pauwels and AO/OTA classification system.

In a recent survey of 298 orthopedic surgeons, 72% preferred the Garden system, only few used the Pauwels (4%) or the AO/OTA (9%).[64] Only 39% of the surveyed surgeons believed that they could distinguish all the four Garden types of fractures, while 96% felt that they could distinguish displaced from undisplaced fractures.[64] These findings may contribute to poor inter and intra-observer reliability of the Garden system as reported in literature. Several authors have suggested abandoning the Gardens system in favor of simpler classification of displaced vs undisplaced fractures.

SURGICAL FIXATION DOES TIMING MATTER?

Significant controversy exists in literature related to optimal timing of surgery for hip fractures in the elderly. For obvious reasons delay in surgery is avoided as for as possible. Incidences of complications and adverse psychological impact on the elderly patient are higher. In 31 studies investigating the impact of surgical delay on mortality rates, 13 studies showed no difference in mortality related to delay in treatment while 18 studies reported increased mortality related to delayed surgical treatment.[61-63] Interestingly all studies that show no difference in mortality following delayed surgery continue to follow the principle of surgery within 24-48 hours. All these studies have based their recommendation on the fact that although no significant difference in mortality was found related to surgical timing, early surgery was associated with shorter hospital stay, less complications, pressure sores, significantly reduced pain and earlier return to independent living.

Based on current level II and level III evidence, we recommend surgical intervention within 24-48 hours to minimize postoperative complications and reduce mortality rates.

TREATMENT

Elderly patients in whom a femoral neck fracture is diagnosed are ideally managed surgically with the aim of return to the preoperative ambulatory and functional status.

A hip fracture is probably the most feared and devastating consequence of osteoporosis in the increasing elderly population. Even after modern treatment, the individual patient has an increased mortality risk and is likely to experience a major negative impact on hip function and quality of life. The ideal treatment of hip fractures is still controversial, more so from an international perspective. One reason for the long-lasting controversy regarding the optimal treatment for the elderly patients may be explained by the ambition to find a single surgical method to treat all patients with a displaced fracture of the femoral neck. During the last decade, several studies have indicated the importance of a treatment algorithm based upon the patient's age, functional demands, pre-fracture walking ability, cognitive function, fracture type and risk factors. However, the population of elderly patients with femoral neck fractures comprises several subpopulations with different functional demands, risk factors and life expectancies. Furthermore, the surgical treatment of displaced femoral neck fractures differs from the treatment of many other hip fractures because the available treatment modalities differ regarding surgical impact, rehabilitation, complications and the long-term outcome. However, optimizing the treatment for improved outcomes and a reduced need for secondary surgery is mandatory for humanitarian and economical needs. The treatment of femoral neck fractures in the mobile elderly is thus directed at rapid restoration of pre-injury functional and ambulatory status.[10,11]

There is a high reported perioperative mortality rate in this elderly population, ranging from 2.4% to 8.2% at one month (Parvizi et al. 2001, Radcliff et al. 2008) and over 25% at one year (Elliott et al. 2003, Jiang et al. 2005).[12]

Conservative treatment is fraught with the complications of prolonged recumbence including chest and urinary infections, pressure sores and disuse osteoporosis. Non-operative management may be preferable for non-ambulatory, institutionalized patients with marked dementia who experience minimal discomfort within the first few days after the injury. Such patient's "return to pre-injury level of function" is better accomplished without surgery. However, early mobilization is essential to avoid the associated complications. The number of patients falling into this category is usually quite small.[13]

External fixation for cervicotrochanteric fractures is another minimally invasive technique available. In elderly patients who are unfit to undergo open surgery, external fixation can be done under local anesthesia and image control. It is a short procedure that aids in early mobilization and nursing care of the patient and avoids complications associated with anaesthesia and prolonged recumbence.

The accepted consensus amongst surgeons worldwide regarding the treatment of undisplaced fractures (garden type 1 and 2) which constitute about 30% of femoral neck fractures is using internal fixation, however the optimal choice for treatment of displaced fractures remains controversial.

INTERNAL FIXATION

Failed Internal Fixation for Fracture Neck Femur

Internal fixation (IF) of femoral neck fractures is either with cannulated cancellous screws or a hip screw with a sliding plate. Parker et al. in a review of

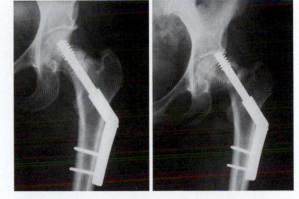

Figure 2: Failed internal fixation for fracture neck femur

displaced femoral neck fractures stated that for those aged less than 50-60 years, preservation of femoral head is of paramount importance.[14] With advancing age the argument against arthroplasty diminishes since the life expectancy of the patient becomes less than the life expectancy of the implant and the functional demands on the hip are less (Figure 2).

Among elderly patients with displaced fractures, the rate of fracture-healing complications after IF is considerably higher, being, in most studies with an at least 2-year follow-up, in the range of 35-50%.[15-17] These failures are more common in patients with displaced fractures, significant osteoporosis and advanced age. Moreover, many patients experience impaired hip function and a reduced health-related quality of life (HRQoL) despite an uneventfully healed fracture.[18] Less or minimally invasive hardware insertion techniques have been shown to reduce transfusion rates, but have no impact on mortality. Anatomic reduction and adequate cortical support are of paramount importance to avoid a secondary loss of reduction.

Fracture healing complications in elderly patients treated with IF are usually divided into non-union (including early redisplacement or progressive displacement with implant failure/cutout) and avascular necrosis (AVN). The follow-up period has to be at least two years to reveal the majority of the fracture healing complications. However, AVN may occur even later, at least up to four years after the fracture.[19] The number of secondary arthroplasties after failed

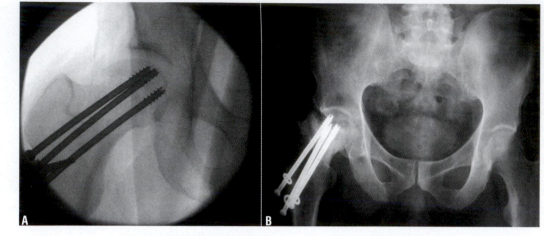

Figures 3A and B: (A) Multiple screw fixation; (B) Failed fixation

internal fixation are nearly always relative and must be balanced against surgical risks. This decision differs between surgeons and because of local therapeutic traditions and resources. Furthermore, it has been shown that a secondary arthroplasty after failed IF will result in inferior hip function compared to a primary arthroplasty.[5,20] According to a prospective randomized comparative study by Keating et al. which compared the treatment of displaced femoral neck fractures in the elderly with internal fixation, hemi-arthroplasty or total hip arthroplasty, it was found that the internal fixation procedure was associated with high rates of revision surgery and an inferior functional outcome compared with that of arthroplasty. This trend was particularly evident in patients aged 60-74 years and older. Although the reduction and internal fixation group had the lowest acute-admission costs (with less expensive implants, shorter operative time and shorter hospital stay), the greatly increased need for re-admissions and re-operations result in this management option having the highest costs overall (Figures 3A and B).[21]

Internal fixation has been relatively uncontroversial in the treatment of undisplaced (Garden I and II) femoral neck fractures even in elderly osteoporotic patients. Among patients with undisplaced fractures, the rate of fracture healing complications after IF is in the range of 5-10% in most studies and good results regarding function and the health-related quality of

life (HRQoL) can be expected 4. The opinion that this outcome is good has recently been challenged by Rogmark et al. in a study including 224 consecutive patients with undisplaced femoral neck fractures treated with IF, in which 40% of the patients stated that they had pain while walking and 9% needed a secondary arthroplasty.

Blomfeldt et al.[60] randomly allocated 102 patients older than 70 years with independent living status and displaced femoral neck fractures to THA vs internal fixation. Four years after the index procedure, complications were found to be 4% in the THA cohort vs 42% in the internal fixation group, and re-operations were necessary in 4% of the THA group vs 47% of the internal fixation cohort.

ARTHROPLASTY

Prosthetic replacement has increasingly become a better option for displaced intra-capsular fracture neck of the femur, especially in elderly patients. The various options available have been the unipolar hemi-arthroplasty, bipolar hemi-arthroplasty and total hip replacement. The use of these options varies considerably among different surgeons and centers. Each option has advantages and disadvantages. It is clear that a patient with antecedent symptomatic osteoarthritis or inflammatory arthritis of the hip, who subsequently suffers a displaced sub-capital hip fracture, would benefit most from a total hip replacement compared to a hemi-arthroplasty.[22] In addition; a patient who suffers a pathological femoral neck fracture with concomitant acetabular pathology should have a total hip replacement performed. When choosing between total hip and hemiarthroplasty, it has been shown that total hip arthroplasty gives a better functional outcome in the elderly, but with higher rate of dislocation.[22] Hemi-arthroplasty results in fewer dislocations, a shorter operating time and less need for blood transfusions, but with a risk that acetabular erosion that might limit the pain-free life of the implant.[22] A bipolar hemi-arthroplasty has the potential advantage of reducing the risk of acetabular wear for patients with a life expectancy of more than five years. On the other hand, a potential disadvantage is the risk of polyethylene wear that may contribute to mechanical loosening in a longer time perspective and there is also a risk of interprosthetic dissociation in certain bipolar HAs necessitating open reduction. However, dissociation appears to be rare in modern bipolar surgical systems. For those aged over 80 years or who are inactive, the bipolar joint is probably of some benefit. Its disadvantages include that it is expensive with a rate of dislocation similar to that of unipolar hemiarthroplasty where closed reduction may not be possible in the event of a dislocation episode.[14]

In the treatment of patients with femoral neck fractures most orthopedic surgeons select prosthetic designs that are intended to be used with bone cement. This selection is in conformity with a current meta-analysis stating that a cemented prosthesis is the recommended treatment with less reported pain and better walking ability compared to uncemented prostheses.[23] However, the frequently used Austin Moore HA (Figures 5A and B) from the 1950s, which is designed for insertion without cement, was used in a number of the studies included in the meta-analysis and an additional conclusion[23] is that this prosthesis should not be used due to inferior results.[23] In a study by Figved et al.[24] included 220 patients randomized to a cemented bipolar hemiarthroplasty or a hydroxyapatite-coated bipolar hemiarthroplasty, the results showed essentially comparable outcomes for all the outcome measures studied, but there were

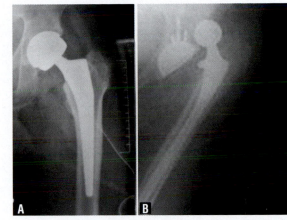

Figures 4A and B: (A) THR; (B) Dislocated THR

6% of intraoperative and postoperative periprosthetic fractures in the uncemented group compared to 2% in the cemented group. However, no cement-related complications were recorded.

TOTAL HIP ARTHROPLASTY VS BIPOLAR HEMIARTHROPLASTY (FIGURES 4A AND B)

In a study of 166 patients who were managed for acute femoral neck fractures with either hemi-arthroplasty or total hip replacement, Gebhard et al. found that the perioperative rate of complications was comparable for the two procedures but total hip replacement resulted in better relief of pain and better function.[25]

Dorr in a study of 89 patients with an acute fracture of the femoral neck who had been randomized to either a total hip arthroplasty or hemi-arthroplasty (with or without cement) found more perioperative complications (mostly dislocations) in the group that had a total hip arthroplasty.[26] However, patients who had a high level of activity had better relieve of pain and better function after total hip replacement when compared to those who had a hemi-arthroplasty.

The potential advantage of using total hip replacement relates to its highly predictable results, with survivorship of greater than 90% at 10 years and its unparalleled results in terms of pain relief and overall function. In addition, the use of total hip replacement avoids the potential need for revision secondary to acetabular pain from ongoing acetabular erosion.[24]

The potential disadvantages include the increased cost, increased surgical time and blood loss (which may lead to increased morbidity or mortality) and the potential increased rate of dislocation compared to hemi-arthroplasty. In Scandinavia, where total hip replacement is commonly used to treat hip fractures, several studies reporting on patients with displaced sub-capital hip fractures randomized to receive either internal fixation or some form of arthroplasty (hemi or total) have concluded that the overall re-operation rate was significantly less and general function was considerably better in those patients receiving a total hip arthroplasty.[27-30] The rate of dislocation ranged from 2-22% (comparable to the dislocation rate of 5.3% in total hip series) and was linked to both the surgical approach and the mental status of the patient.[27-30] What remains unclear is whether certain hip fracture patients, with no pre-existing hip pathology, would benefit from total hip replacement rather than hemi-arthroplasty. Rogmark et al. have suggested that patients between the ages of 70-80 years are the ideal candidates for total hip replacement.[28] In contrast; patients who are greater than 80 years of age are best treated with hemi-arthroplasty.

There are more and more data indicating that ambulant elderly patients with a displaced fracture of the femoral neck should be treated with a primary hip arthroplasty.[31,32] The most recent Cochrane review with the latest update in December 2009, 25 presented four studies comparing cemented HA with THA.[28-30] The meta-analysis showed a trend towards better functional outcome after THA, but no conclusion could be drawn because of insufficient power and further randomized trials with an adequate length of follow-up were recommended.

In clinical practice, the opinion among orthopedic surgeons seems to be that HA is the preferred treatment for elderly patients with low functional demands, while the choice of arthroplasty type for healthy, active, elderly patients is more controversial. The most common complication after THA in patients with femoral neck fracture has been dislocation of the prosthesis, which may be one reason why some surgeons hesitate to perform a primary THA. However, recent studies have shown that utilization of an anterolateral approach and judicious patient selection can reduce the dislocation rate to a level at a par with that expected after THA in patients with arthritic hips, i.e. 0- 2%.[33,34] Of special interest regarding the choice of HA versus THA are also data from studies with longer follow-up times including active patients treated with a primary HA. In active patients there are potential problems of acetabular erosion which may result in impaired hip function and the need for revision arthroplasty.

A published study comparison between bipolar HA and THA included 138 patients and the 2-year results for THA appeared to be better than those for bipolar HA. Baker et al.[35] compared a cemented unipolar HA with a cemented THA in 81 patients. The functional outcome, based on the Oxford hip score and self reported walking distance, significantly favored the THA group, while the HRQoL according to SF-3668 did not differ significantly between the groups.

After the latest update of the Cochrane review in December 2009, 2 additional RCTs comparing HA and THA have been published. The study by Macaulay and Coworkers included 40 patients randomized to either HA (unipolar or bipolar) or THA. Although the overall results for hip function, as assessed by HHS and WOMAC and HRQoL were in favor of the THA group, the differences were not statistically significant, most probably due to a lack of study power. However, some of the subscores, such as the WOMAC and the SF-36, were reported to be significantly better in the THA group.[36]

In 2010 Bekerom et al. reported the 5-year outcome for patients randomized to treatment with a THA or a bipolar HA. The overall conclusion of the study differs markedly from other RCTs. Because of a higher intraoperative blood loss, an increased duration of the operation, and a higher number of early and late dislocations, the authors do not recommend THA as the treatment of choice in patients aged > 70 years with a fracture of the femoral neck. The overall dislocation rate in the THA group was as high as 7%, which may be explained by the use of the posterolateral approach in almost 20% of the patients. The dislocation rate among those operated upon via an anterolateral approach was

1% compared to 19% among those operated upon using a posterolateral approach. It has been shown that dislocations, especially recurrent ones, have a negative influence on the patients' perception of their quality of life due to their impaired hip function.

There were an increased number of hip complications in the THA group: 3 compared to 1. However, 2 of these complications, the periprosthetic fracture and the late hematogenous infection, could not be related to the surgical method per se, while, theoretically, the early deep infection could be related to the fact that THA is a slightly more time-consuming surgical procedure.[37]

HEMIARTHROPLASTY-UNIPOLAR OR BIPOLAR?

Hemiarthroplasty is considered the optimal treatment for elderly patients with displaced femoral neck fractures, and produces satisfactory results. Nonetheless, for older patients who are mobile, socially independent and fit, the treatment is controversial. Internal fixation has a high rate of nonunion and is inferior to hemiarthroplasty. According to the Norwegian Hip Fracture Register, patients treated with hemiarthroplasty had less pain and were more satisfied with the outcome than those treated with internal fixation.[38] In a recent international survey questionnaire sent to 442 orthopedic surgeons, 94-96% preferred a hip arthroplasty for a patient aged 80 years or more with a Garden type III or IV fracture.

The choice was a unipolar HA in 60% and a bipolar HA in 32-33%.[39] However, the choice between a unipolar and a bipolar HA is controversial and difficult to make. Bipolar prostheses enable reduction of acetabular wear and increase in prosthesis life and function. Compared to unipolar hemiarthroplasty, bipolar hemiarthroplasty confers better or similar overall outcomes as well as better pain relief and function. It is therefore recommended for active elderly patients. Although bipolar prostheses are more costly, they may be cost-effective given their effects on outcomes. For patients aged 60-80 years with displaced femoral neck fractures, bipolar hemiarthroplasty is most commonly used, whereas for those aged >80 years, unipolar hemiarthroplasty was more popular. There is no definite cut-off age for unipolar or bipolar hemiarthroplasty. The Scottish intercollegiate guidelines 2 and other studies recommend cemented hemiarthroplasty.[40] Cemented bipolar hemiarthroplasty achieves good short-and long-term results.[40]

Active elderly patients (aged 70-90 years) with femoral neck fractures have poor results after unipolar hemiarthroplasty owing to increased demands on such a hip and consequent acetabular erosion (Figures 6A and B). Acetabular erosion appeared to have a significant negative effect on functional outcome and HRQoL

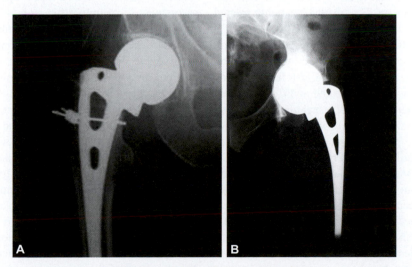

Figures 5A and B: Austin Moore arthroplasty

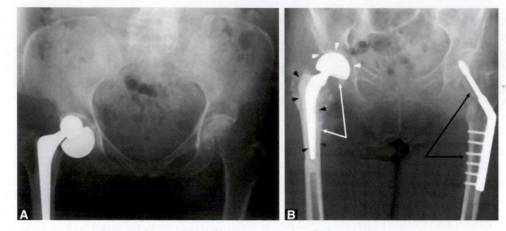

Figures 6A and B: (A) Disloacated bipolar; (B) Acetabular erosion

The results of most RCT have not demonstrate much differences regarding complications, hip function and HRQoL in elderly patients with a displaced fracture of the femoral neck randomized to either a unipolar HA or a bipolar HA. However, after one year, radiological signs of acetabular erosion were significantly more frequent after the unipolar HA than the bipolar HA.

Acetabular erosion has been considered to be one important factor for impaired hip function and in previous reports, the rate of acetabular erosion has ranged from 12 to 36% for unipolar designs and from 10 to 26% for bipolar designs.[41] Baker et al. reported acetabular erosion in 21 out of 32 patients treated with a unipolar HA after a mean follow-up of 39 months, giving an overall rate of acetabular erosion of 66%.[42] This opinion is supported by the study by D'Arcy and Devas 77 including 361 femoral neck fractures in 354 patients treated with a cemented unipolar HA where the rate of acetabular erosion was highest and the clinical results worst in the younger patients.

There are studies on earlier designs of the bipolar prosthesis showing that the bipolar HA already functions as a unipolar HA a few months (3-12) after surgery, but recent studies display a significantly higher rate of acetabular erosion in the unipolar HA group, indicate that there is a real advantage in favor of the bipolar design, which is most probably due to the function of the dual-bearing system.

THE SEVERELY COGNITIVELY IMPARED PATIENT INTERNAL FIXATION VS HEMOARTHROPLASTY

Delirium (i.e. acute confusion) and dementia are two well-known risk factors in the treatment of hip fracture patients. A common denominator of both these conditions is the presence of cognitive dysfunction, defined as a disturbance in the patient's mental processes related to thinking, reasoning and judgment. Previous studies indicate that hip fracture patients with impaired cognitive function have an increased risk for general as well as fracture-related complications.[24] Despite this knowledge, an assessment of cognitive function is often lacking in nursing and medical records for a substantial number of older people with hip fractures.[43,44] Patients with severe cognitive dysfunction pose significant challenges to the treating surgeon in several respects, e.g. lack of compliance, problems in assimilating rehabilitation procedures, frequent falls and co-morbidities. In patients with an associated displaced femoral neck fracture, this may severely affect the outcome after a hip arthroplasty, as shown in the study by Johansson et al. in which the dislocation rate after a THR was 32% in cognitively impaired patients.[45] In one previous study including severely cognitively impaired patients with displaced femoral neck fractures, sixty patients were randomized to either IF or HA (Figures 5A and B) (uncemented Austin Moore, prosthesis). The one-year mortality rate was

43% and the two-year rate was 57%. Functional outcome was reported at the one year follow-up and among one year survivors who were walkers before the fracture; only 20% in the HA group and 36% in the IF group were still mobile. There were wound infections in 17% in the HA group and deep infections requiring surgical intervention in at least 3.4%. The general conclusion was that the chance of successful rehabilitation was small regardless of the surgical procedure and that IF was the treatment of choice because it is a minor surgical procedure with less morbidity.

CEMENTED VS CEMENTLESS ARTHROPLASTY

Cemented Hemi- or total hip arthroplasty is an established treatment for femoral neck fracture in the mobile elderly. Cemented prostheses have been used with high success rates in the past.[46,47] It has been reported to be associated with relatively fewer complications and low mortality rates. Elderly frail patients tolerate bone cement as it reinforces osteoporotic proximal femurs.[46] Cemented femoral component provides an immediate postoperative advantage, i.e. of intimate contact between the prosthesis cement and the bone, which permits dramatic early relief of pain and early and more weight-bearing. Literature review shows that for a short-term outcome, almost all the relevant studies reported superiority of the cemented fixation to the uncemented in terms of pain reduction, thigh pain, hip score, walking with support, gait analysis, etc. Moreover, periprosthetic femoral fractures that have been reported with cementless hemiarthroplasty are less common with cemented stems.[46]

In 2002, Khan et al. conducted a systematic review on whether better outcomes could be achieved by cemented hemiarthroplasty in treating patients with displaced intracapsular femoral neck fractures. They concluded that the literature tended to support the use of cement.[48]

A Cochrane database survey,[49] with 17 trials involving 1920 patients, confirmed that with cemented prostheses patients had less pain, better mobility and no significant difference in complications compared with cementless prostheses patients, at a mean follow-up of one year. Similarly, no significant differences were found between unipolar and bipolar hemiarthroplasty (seven trials, 857 participants, 863 fractures).[49] Dorr et al.[50] also, in his prospective study of treatment of displaced femoral neck fractures found no differences in pain, ambulation or aids required between any of the femoral stem fixation methods. They advised against the use of cementless femoral stems in wide canals (Dorr type C and D femurs) due to higher instances of subsidence and loosening as a result of inadequate press-fit.[49]

Postoperative mortality following hip replacements is usually due to cardiopulmonary causes (myocardial infarction or pulmonary emboli).[49] Intraoperative deaths (cardiac arrest) during hip arthroplasty occur infrequently and have been associated with bone cement (BCIS).[51] Patients with severe underlying cardiovascular disease are more prone to this problem.[51] The hemodynamic effects of medullary fat embolism during the process of cement pressurization rather than the toxic effects of the cement itself cause BCIS. Rarely, this syndrome may occur in the absence of methyl methacrylate use.[50] As reported by Lo and Chen, cemented replacements require relatively more time and have more blood loss as compared to cementless replacements.[52]

Cementless stems avert this bone cement implantation syndrome (BCIS),[50] though there have been many complications noted with this technique (for example, perioperative fractures, loosening and subsidence with thigh pain).[50] The advantages of the cemented technique seem to be offset by its mortality risk and the advantages of the cementless option by its increased morbidity. Thus, in some of these very elderly morbid patients, the orthopedic surgeon is faced with a dilemma as to the correct surgical choice, which should be one that can promise pain relief and rapid resumption of function and at the same time, reduce mortality and morbidity.

Newer cementing techniques have eliminated many problems associated with earlier fixations, especially better filling of the spaces between the prosthesis and surrounding bone. Using the newest advances in cementing techniques, the Charnley low friction cemented arthroplasty is regarded by many as the standard treatment for comparison purposes

OSTEOPOROTIC FEMORAL NECK FRACTURES

5. Ali Nawaz Khan, Sumaira Mc Donald osteoporosis, involutional; 2008.

6. Zetterberg C, Elmerson S, Andersson GB. Epidemiology of hip fractures in Goteborg, Sweden, 1940-1983. Clin Orthop; 1984.pp.43-52.

7. Vellas B, Conceicao J, Lafont C, Fontan B, Garry PJ, Adoue D, et al. Malnutrition and falls. Lancet 1990;336:1447.

8. Lotz JC, Hayes WC. The use of quantitative computed tomography to estimate risk of fracture of the hip from falls. J Bone Joint Surg [Am] 1990;72:689-700.

9. Lumbars M, Driver LT, Howland RJ, Older MWJ, Williams CM. Nutritional status and clinical outcome in elderly female surgical orthopaedic patients. Clinical Nutrition; 1996.pp.101-7.

10. Dorr LD, Glousman R, Hoy AL, Vanis R, Chandler R. Treatment of femoral neck fractures with total hip replacement versus cemented and noncemented hemiarthroplasty. J Arthroplasty 1986; 1:21-8.

11. Leighton RK, Schmidt AH, Collier P, Trask K. Advances in the treatment of intracapsular hip fractures in the elderly. Injury 2007;38:S24-34

12. Darren J Costainl, Sarah L Whitehousel, Nicole L Pratt, Stephen E Graves4, Philip Ryan3, and Ross W Crawford Perioperative mortality after hemiarthroplasty related to fixation method. Ada Orthopaedica 2011; 82 (3): 275-81.

13. Holmberg S, Kalen R, Thorngren KG. Treatment and outcome of femoral neck fractures: An analysis of 2418 patients admitted from their own homes. Clin Orthop Relat Res 1987;218:42-52.

14. Parker MJ. The management of intracapsular fractures of the proximal femur. J Bone Joint Surg Br 200;82:937-41.

15. Trueta J, Harrison MHM. The normal vascular anatomy of the femoral head in adult man. J Bone Joint Surg Br 1953;35:442-460.

16. Weigl M, Cieza A, Cantista P, Reinhardt JD, stucki G. Determinants of disability in chronic muscul-oskeletal health conditions: A literature review. Eur General phys rehabil Med. 2008; 44(2):67-9.

17. Pauwels F. Der Schenkelhalsborch; Ein Mechan-isches problem. Stuttgart: Ferdinand Enke Verlag; 1935.

18. Gaden RS. Malreduction and avascular necrosis in subcapital fractures of the femur. J bone Joint Surg Br 1971;53:183-96.

19. Lowell JD. Fractures of the hip. N England J Med 1966;274:1418-25.

20. Bayliss AP, Davison JK. Traumatic osteonecrosis of the femoral head following intracapsular fracture: incidence and earliest radiological features. Clinradiol 1977;28:407-14.

21. Keating JF, Grant A, Masson M, Scott NW, Forbes JF. Randomized comparison of reduction and fixation, bipolar hemiarthroplasty and total hip arthroplasty in the treatment of displaced intracapsular hip fractures in healthy older patients. J Bone Joint Surg Am 2006;88:249-60.

22. Squires B, Bannister G. Displaced intracapsular neck of femur fractures in mobile independent patients: Total hip replacement or hemiarthroplasty? Injury 1999;30:345-8.

23. Parker MJ, Gurusamy KS, Azegami S. Arthroplasties (with and without bone cement) for proximal femoral fractures in adults. Cochrane Database Syst Rev 2010;6:CD001706.

24. Figved W, Opland V, Frihagen F, Jervidalo T, Madsen JE, Nordsletten L. Cemented versus uncemented hemiarthroplasty for displaced femoral neck fractures. Clin Orthop Relat Res 2009 Sep; 467(9):2426-35.

25. Parker MJ, Gurusamy KS, Azegami S. Arthroplasties (with and without bone cement) for proximal femoral fractures in adults. Cochrane Database Syst Rev 2010;6:CD001706.

26. Varley J, Parker MJ. Stability of hip hemiar-throplasties. Int Orthop 2004;28(5):274-7.

27. Skinner P, Riley D, Ellery J, Beaumont A, Coumine R, Shafighian B. Displaced subcapital fractures of the femur: a prospective randomized comparison of internal fixation, hemiarthroplasty and total hip replacement. Injury 1989;20(5):291-3.

28. Blomfeldt R, Tornkvist H, Eriksson K, Soderqvist A, Ponzer S, Tidermark J. A randomised controlled trial comparing bipolar hemiarthroplasty with total hip replacement for displaced intracapsular fractures of the femoral neck in elderly patients. J Bone Joint Surg Br 2007;89(2):160-5.57.

29. Baker RP, Squires B, Gargan MF, Bannister GC. Total hip arthroplasty and hemiarthroplasty in mobile, independent patients with a displaced intracapsular fracture of the femoral neck. A randomized, controlled trial. J Bone Joint Surg Am 2006;88(12):2583-9.

30. Dorr LD, Glousman R, Hoy AL, Vanis R, Chandler R. Treatment of femoral neck fractures with total hip replacement versus cemented and noncemented hemiarthroplasty. J Arthroplasty 1986;l(1):21-8.

31. Blomfeldt R, Tornkvist H, Ponzer S, Soderqvist A, Tidermark J. Comparison of internal fixation with total hip replacement for displaced femoral neck

fractures. Randomized, controlled trial performed at four years. J Bone Joint Surg Am 2005;87(8): 1680-8.

32. Rogmark C, Carlsson A, Johnell O, Sernbo I. A prospective randomised trial of internal fixation versus arthroplasty for displaced fractures of the neck of the femur. Functional outcome for 450 patients at two years. J Bone Joint Surg Br 2002; 84(2): 183-8.

33. Tidermark J, Ponzer S, Svensson O, Soderqvist A, Tornkvist H. Internal fixation compared with total hip replacement for displaced femoral neck fractures in the elderly. A randomised, controlled trial. J Bone Joint Surg Br 2003;85(3):380-8.

34. Enocson A, Tidermark J, Tornkvist H, Lapidus LJ. Dislocation of hemiarthroplasty after femoral neck fracture: better outcome after the anterolateral approach in a prospective cohort study on 739 consecutive hips. Acta Orthop 2008;79(2):211-7.

35. Baker RP, Squires B, Gargan MF, Bannister GC. Total hip arthroplasty and hemiarthroplasty in mobile, independent patients with a displaced intracapsular fracture of the femoral neck. A randomized, controlled trial. J Bone Joint Surg Am 2006;88(12):2583-9.

36. Macaulay W, Nellans KW, Garvin KL, Iorio R, Healy WL, Rosenwasser MP. Prospective randomized clinical trial comparing hemiarthroplasty to total hip arthroplasty in the treatment of displaced femoral neck fractures: winner of the Dorr Award. J Arthroplasty. 2008;23(6 Suppl l):2-8.

37. van den Bekerom MP, Hilverdink EF, Sierevelt IN, Reuling EM, Schnater JM, Bonke H, et al. A comparison of hemiarthroplasty with total hip replacement for displaced intracapsular fracture of the femoral neck: a randomised controlled multi-centre trial in patients aged 70 years and over. J Bone Joint Surg Br 2010;92(10):422-8.

38. Gjertsen JE, Vinje T, Lie SA, Engesaeter LB, Havelin LI, Fumes O, et al. Patient satisfaction, pain, and quality of life four months after displaced femoral neck fractures: a comparison of 663 fractures treated with internal fixation and 906 with bipolar hemiarthroplasty reported to the Norwegian Hip Fracture Register. Acta Orthop 2008;79:(5)94-601.

39. Bhandari M, Devereaux PJ, Tometta P, Swiontkowski MF, Berry DJ, Haidukewych G, et al. Operative management of displaced femoral neck fractures in elderly patients: an international survey 3rd edition. J Bone Joint Surg Am 2005;87(9):2122-30.

40 Huo MH, Gilbert NF. What's new in hip arthroplasty. J Bone Joint Surg Am 2005;87:2133-46.

41 Squires B, Bannister G. Displaced intracapsular neck of femur fractures in mobile independent patients: total hip replacement or hemiarthroplasty? Injury. 1999;30(5): 345-8.

42. Baker RP, Squires B, Gargan MF, Bannister GC. Total hip arthroplasty and hemiarthroplasty in mobile, independent patients with a displaced intracapsular fracture of the femoral neck. A randomized, controlled trial. J Bone Joint Surg Am. 2006;88(12):2583-9.

43. Gustafson Y, Brannstrom B, Norberg A, Bucht G, Winblad B. Underdiagnosis and poor documentation of acute confusional states in elderly hip fracture patients. J Am Geriatr Soc 1991;39:760-5.

44. Soderqvist A, Miedel R, Ponzer S, Tidermark J. The influence of cognitive function on outcome after a hip fracture. J Bone Joint Surg Am 2006;88:2115-23.

45. Johansson T, Jacobsson SA, Ivarsson I, Knutsson A, Wahlstrom O. Internal fixation versus total hip arthroplasty in the treatment of displaced femoral neck fractures: a prospective randomized study of 100 hips. Acta Orthop Scand 2000;71:597-602.

46. Lo WH, Chen WM, Huang CK, Chen TH, Chiu FY, Chen CM. Bateman bipolar hemiarthroplasty for displaced intracapsular femoral neck fractures: Uncemented versus cemented. Clin Orthop Relat Res 1994;302:75-82

47. Ozturkmen Y, Karamehmetoglu M, Caniklioglu M, Ince Y, Azboy Y. Cementless hemiarthroplasty for femoral neck fractures in elderly patients. Indian J Orthop 2008;42(1):56-60

48. Khan RJ, MacDowell A, Crossman P, Keene GS. Cemented or uncemented hemiarthroplasty for displaced intracapsular fractures of the hip—a systematic review. Injury 2002;33:13-7.

49. Parker MJ, Gurusamy K. Arthroplasties (with and without bone cement) for proximal femoral fractures in adults. Cochrane Database Syst Rev 2006;3:CD001706.

50. Dorr LD, Glousman R, Hoy AL, Vanis R, Chandler R. Treatment of femoral neck fractures with total hip replacement versus cemented and noncemented hemiarthroplasty. J Arthroplasty 1986; 1:21-8.

51. Parvizi J, Holiday AD, Ereth MH, Lewallen DG. Sudden death during primary hip arthroplasty. Clin Orthop Relat Res 1999;369:39-48.

52. Lo WH, Chen WM, Huang CK, Chen TH, Chiu FY, Chen CM. Bateman bipolar hemiarthroplasty for displaced intracapsular femoral neck fractures: Uncemented versus cemented. Clin Orthop Relat Res 1994;302:75-82

53. Pieringer H, Labek G, Auersperg V, Bohler N. Cementless total hip arthroplasty in patients older than 80 years of age. J Bone Joint Surg Br 2003;85:641-5.

54. Wykman A, Olsson E, Axdorph G, Goldie I. Total hip arthroplasty. A comparison between cemented and press-fit noncemented fixation. J Arthroplasty 1991;6:19-29.

55. Godsiff SP, Emery RJ, Heywood-Waddington MB, Thomas TL. Cemented versus uncemented femoral components in the ring hip prosthesis. J Bone Joint Surg Br l992;74:822-4.

56. Emerson RH Jr, Head WC, Emerson CB, Rosenfeldt W, Higgins LL. A comparison of cemented and cementless titanium femoral components used for primary total hip arthroplasty: a radiographic and survivorship study. J Arthroplasty 2002;17:584-91.

57. Havelin LI, Espehaug B, Vollset SE, Engesaeter LB. The effect of the type of cement on early revision of Charnley total hip prostheses. A review of eight thousand five hundred and seventy-nine primary arthroplasties from the Norwegian Arthroplasty Register. J Bone Joint Surg Am 1995;77:1543-50.

58. Kirk PG, Rorabeck CH, Bourne RB, Burkart B. Total hip arthroplasty in rheumatoid arthritis: comparison of cemented and uncemented implants. Can J Surg 1993;36: 229-32.

59. Knessl J, Gschwend N, Scheier H, Munzinger U. Comparative study of cemented and cementless hip prostheses in the same patient. Arch Orthop Trauma Surg 1989; 108:276-8.

60. Blomfeldt R, Tomkvist H, Ponzer S, Soderqvist A. Tidermark J. Comparison of internal fixation with total hip replacement for displaced femoral neck fractures. Randomized, controlied trial performed at four years. J Bone Joint Swn Am 2005;87(8):1680-88.

61. Elliott J, Beringer T, Kee F, Marsh D, Willis C, Stevenson M. Predicting survival after treatment for fracture of the proximal femur and the effect of delaystosurgery. J Cliri Epidemiol 2003;56(S): 7S8-795.

62. Orosz GM, Magaziner J, Hannan EL. et ai. Association of timing of surgery for hip fracture and patient outcomes. JAMA 2004;291(14):1738-43.

63. Ai-Ani AN. Samuelsson B, Tidermark J, et al. Early operation on patients with a hip fracture improved the ability to return to independent iivinq. A prospective study of 850 patients. J Bone Joint Sum Am 2008; 90(7):1436-42.

64. Ziowodzki M, Bhandari M, Keel M, Hanson BP, Schemitsch E. Perception of Garden's classification for femoral neck fractures; an international survey of 298 orthopaedic trauma surgeons. Arch Orthop Trauma Surg 2005;125(7):503-5.

8 | An Overview of Total Hip Arthroplasty in Rheumatoid Arthritis

SV Vaidya, Sachin G Gujarathi, Arvind Arora

Rheumatoid arthritis (RA) is a multisystemic inflammatory disorder affecting bone and joints.It is known since ancient times as described in *Charak Samhita*, though the term Rheumatoid arthritis was coined in 18th century by Alfred Baring Garrod.[1] It affects 3/10,000 population with female preponderance in age group of 35 to 50 years.[2-4]

Management of rheumatoid arthritis involves a multidisciplinary approach involving rheumatologist, physician, chest physician, physical therapist, orthotist, orthopedic and arthroplasty surgeons in synchronization at different stages of disease. Orthopedic surgeon has a major role in management at every stage of the disease, viz. synovitis, arthritis, fibrous ankylosis, bony ankylosis.

It predominantly affects small joints. However hip affection is seen in up to 20% of the cases with 3% having severe destructive pattern.[3] Rheumatoid arthritis has tendency towards symmetrical involvement. Simultaneous hip and knee affection can be encountered posing challenging situation, more so if associated with deformities and stiffness. It requires careful planning based on experience and aimed at the overall management of patient rather than focus only on joint replacement to alleviate disability.

Total hip arthroplasty is an accepted treatment modality for sequelae of this disease; say arthritis, ankylosis, protrusio acetabuli, avascular necrosis of hip and fracture neck femur. It reduces the disability significantly and improves the quality of life where other conservative measures fail. However arthroplasty in rheumatoid arthritis needs special considerations in view of difficult anesthesia and its complications, multisystemic involvement with associated comorbidities, adverse effects of medications, osteoporosis and complex acetabular configurations leading to higher chances of local as well as systemic complications.[5-7]

Anesthesia in rheumatoid and other inflammatory arthritis is a skillful task in view of spinal deformities, difficult intubation due to atlantoaxial and subaxial instability of cervical spine, stiffness of temporomandibular joint sometimes requiring nasal intubation or awake intubation while induction.[5-7] Also ischemic heart disease and increased tendency for cardiac failure remains matter of concern in perioperative period.[5,6,8]

Intraoperative blood loss is usually higher owing to increased vascularity due to inflammation. These patients have chronic anemia along with low erythropoietin as well as lower protein levels. All these with cardiac comorbidities necessitate blood conservation techniques to be implemented intraoperatively.[5,9]

Osteoporosis is a matter of concern with rheumatoid arthritis in view of higher chances of intraoperative and postoperative fractures including periprosthetic fractures. Inflammation itself causes osteoporosis in addition to medications like steroids, which along with reduced activity levels aggravate the condition.

Arthroplasty surgeons may encounter complex acetabular configurations intraoperatively which requires technical expertise to manage. Acetabular configurations in rheumatoid arthritis includes;

chondrolytic type with concentric joint space reduction, protrusio acetabuli and ankylosis either fibrous or bony.

Protrusio acetabuli is seen in 1% of rheumatoid patients. It proposes a challenge at each step of arthroplasty. It necessitates a cautious exposure as the sciatic nerve lies close to greater trochanter. Dislocation of femoral head is extremely difficult in these cases. Preservation of bone if any, over the floor of acetabulum (medial wall) while reaming is the rule. Restoration of center of acetabulum is required to restore hip biomechanics by reconstruction of defect using either bone graft alone or along with antiprotrusio cages/meshes with lateralization of acetabulum.

Ankylosis of hip has its own sets of problems; higher chances of injury to sciatic nerve with exposure, difficult femoral neck cut and difficult reaming due to lack of landmarks for acetabular orientation. Also postoperative there are higher chances of dislocation in view of weak abductors and extensors due to disuse wasting or atrophy.

Rheumatoid affects integumentary system as well causing increased fragility of skin. Also medications lead to poor tendency towards wound healing.[6] Chronic anemia and hypoproteinemias associated with inflammatory process contributes to the same and hence there are increased chances of wound complications in rheumatoid arthritis patients. These patients usually have poor perineal hygiene and increased tendency to develop bedsores.

Taking all these into consideration, it necessitates attention towards detailed perioperative, planning with management protocol of arthroplasty in rheumatoid arthritis patients along with surgical expertise.

Indications: Indications of hip arthroplasty in rheumatoid arthritis are arthritis, protrusio acetabuli, ankylosis and avascular necrosis of head of femur. However infection and medical comorbidities are the only contraindications of surgery.

Preoperative counseling: It is an important aspect of perioperative management. The patient should understand the need of procedure she/he is undergoing, the associated complications and limitations after surgery along with the benefits in terms of improvement in quality of life. Lifestyle modification should be explained owing to limitations postsurgery for long-term successful outcome.

Timing of arthroplasty: Hip arthroplasty is an elective procedure and should be done for above mentioned sequelae of the disease once the conservative management has failed. Detailed medical evaluation and laboratory investigations should be done in advance. However once indicated; surgery should not be delayed for reasons other than optimization of the patient, or else complexity of surgery increases with higher chances of complications.

Preoperative Evaluation and Clinical Examination

The preoperative evaluation should take place in office setting several weeks prior to surgery. It allows sufficient time for multidisciplinary approach towards patients with necessary investigations and optimizing the patient status before the anticipated surgery. The optimal preoperative evaluation and the specific needs in a given patient will depend upon factors, such as patients age and comorbidities, current medications, type of anesthesia, bilateral or unilateral surgery, etc.

Clinical examination: Hip joint should be examined with respect to range of motion, deformities and limb length discrepancy. Simultaneous involvement of knee should be documented if present. Assess the abductor and extensor muscles strength in case of long standing ankylosis of hip.[10] Rule out infection at the proposed surgical site due to previous surgery if any or decubitus ulcers in the vicinity. Dental, gastrointestinal and urological evaluation needs to be done to rule out infective foci.[6] Cardiologist and chest physician evaluation is advisable.[5,6] Anesthesiologist assessment should be done in office setting at least few weeks prior to the planned surgery along with the necessary investigations.

Investigations: Complete hematological investigations and biochemical investigations should be done routinely in all patients. Coagulation profile (if on anticoagulants) is indicated for patients taking anticoagulant medications. Chest roentgenogram, HRCT scan of chest and if required pulmonary function tests are to be done as per chest physician's advice to rule out the restrictive pattern of lung disease.Also ECG, 2D echo and if indicated stress test are to be done. Cervical spine instability is a consistent finding in rheumatoid arthritis patients, thus cervical spine radiographs is mandate.[5]

Protocol for Continuation of DMARDs[11]

When a patient with rheumatoid arthritis undergoes surgery, the major problem is to find a balance between maintaining disease control and avoiding an unfavorable impact on wound healing and postoperative complications on the other hand. Continuing medication may hamper wound healing and predisposes to infections. Discontinuation may lead to disease flare, which may increase the need for corticosteroids for disease control and, furthermore limits mobilization and effective rehabilitation after surgery. A limited number of authors have addressed the question of how to best handle antirheumatic treatment in RA patients undergoing surgery. The main results of the review are summarized in the Table 1.

Preoperative Planning

Preoperative planning is essential so as to ensure availability of proper inventory on the day of surgery depending on type and size of selected implants and to prevent limb length discrepancy. Preoperative planning can prevent limb length discrepancy with accuracy up to 5 mm.[12] Also it ensures surgeons preparedness for anticipated intraoperative difficulties such as complex acetabular configurations and measures to tackle them like keeping bone grafts, acetabular cages, etc. ready if required. In case of both hip and knee requiring arthroplasty, planning sequential procedure with alignment radiographs achieves better lower limb biomechanics. It is adviced to perform hip arthroplasty followed by knee.[7,13] Also planning of simultaneous bilateral hip arthroplasty in single anesthesia or staged bilateral procedure should be done beforehand depending on the comorbidities and investigations in bilateral hip arthritis.

Radiographs: Pelvis with both hips and lateral view should be taken in all cases. Anteroposterior

Table 1: Guidelines for the use of antirheumatic drugs in the perioperative period

Drug	Comments
Methotrexate	May be continued in otherwise healthy individuals
Leflomide	Discontinuation seems problematic due to long half-life
Sulfasalazine, azathioprine	Discontinue on day of surgery, no relevant data
Hydroxychloroquine	Appears to be safe, long half-life
TNF-alpha inhibitors	Only limited data, withhold drug a couple of weeks prior to surgery
Anakinra, rituximab, abatacept	No data available
NSAIDs	To exclude antithrombotic effect withhold drug for 4–5 times the half-life
Aspirin	Discontinue for 7–10 days prior to surgery to avoid inhibition of platelet function. Consider other than anti-inflammatory indications (e.g. coronary heart disease)
Glucocorticoids	Do not discontinue perioperatively. Supplement patients with suspected suppression of HPA axis. Regimen depends on type of procedure

(AP) radiograph should be taken in supine position with limb in 15 to 20 degree of internal rotation, to get plane of femoral neck into parallel orientation relative to cassette and perpendicular to X-ray beam. If internal rotation is not possible as in bilateral hip involvement, posteroanterior (PA view) should be taken in prone position with involved extremity in external rotation. X-ray should be taken in semi-sitting position in case of flexion deformity at hip or knee. Magnification factor should be noted for corrections in measurements done. Lateral X-ray is preferred with patient supine and hip in maximal external rotation. Alignment radiograph is indicated in patients with concomitant hip and knee involvement with/without deformities.

Landmarks: Teardrop is the anatomic landmark of inferomedial aspect of acetabulum. It should be marked on both sides. A line connecting tip of both teardrops is to be drawn along with vertical bisector from each teardrop. Superior aspect of tip of lesser trochanter is to be marked. Line joining both ischial tuberosities is to be drawn.

Signs of protrusio: [14–16]Signs of protrusio acetabuli include the acetabular line crossing Kohler's line by more than 3 mm in men and more than 6 mm in women, teardrop appears to be closed or reversed and center-edge angle of Wieberg greater than 46. However, these lack sensitivity and specificity. Grades of protrusio acetabuli can be assessed by following methods: Sotelo-Garza and Charnley classified the grade on basis of distance between medial wall of acetabulum protruding into pelvis and iliopectineal line (upper margin of superior pubic ramus).[15,17,18]

Grade I: (Mild), 1-5 mm

Grade II: (Moderate), 6-15 mm

Grade III: (Severe) more than 15 mm

Fragmentation, absence of medial wall of acetabulum and difficult delineation of the pelvic brim is considered as Grade III. This is most accepted and widely used grading system by most of the authors.

Kohler's line (ilioischial) method: According to distance between acetabular line (medial wall of acetabulum) and ilioischial line (quadrilateral surface of acetabulum.[18,19] However measurements may vary according to pelvic obliquity.[20]

Grade	Men	Women
I	3-8 mm	6-11 mm
II	8-13 mm	12-17 mm
III	> 13 mm with fragmentation	> 17 mm with fragmentation

Horizontal and vertical coordinate method: Superior as well as medial migration of femoral head can be quantified with respect to X and Y coordinates drawn taking teardrops as reference.[20] However lack of teardrop localization limits the utility of this technique.

Limb length discrepancy should be calculated by comparing vertical distance between biischial line and tip of lesser trochanter on both sides. Document the vertical offset of femur by measuring distance between center of femoral head to tip of lesser trochanter for intraoperative reference.

Type of femoral canal should be distinguished for selection of the implant type and its fixation modality. Dossick et al. classified proximal femoral configuration on basis of calcar : canal ratio. It is calculated by division of outer diameter of femur at mid of lesser trochanter by diameter at a point 10 cm distal.[21]

- Type A: Ratio less than 0.5; thick cortices on both AP and lateral radiographs. Compatible for uncemented femoral component.
- Type B: Ratio 0.5 to 0.75; thinning of posterior cortex on lateral view. Either uncemented or cemented femoral prosthesis can be opted.
- Type C: Ratio more than 0.75; thinning of cortices on both the views. Cemented femoral prosthesis is desirable.

Templating

Acetabular templating: Keep template at 45° inclination just lateral to teardrop on line joining both teardrops. The component size which spans between teardrop and superolateral edge of the acetabulum with minimal removal of subchondral bone should be selected. Two to three millimeter of space should be considered for cement mantle in case of cemented arthroplasty. This is usually indicated by dotted lines on templates. The center of rotation should be marked through template. The horizontal and vertical distance from teardrop to center of rotation is to be compared with corresponding co-ordinates on contralateral unaffected hip.

Ranawat et al. described method for planning of acetabular cup in protrusio. Parallel horizontal lines are to be drawn at level of iliac crest and ischial tuberosities. A perpendicular joining both is to be drawn passing through 5 mm lateral to intersection of Kohler's and Shenton's line. One-fifth of the height of perpendicular between parallel lines approximately corresponds to height of acetabulum. Another perpendicular is drawn from point located at the height of acetabulum on vertical line; it corresponds to superior aspect of subchondral bone of acetabulum. Isosceles triangle is drawn connecting both the perpendiculars with hypotenuse being diameter of acetabular cup for intended reconstruction.[22]

Femoral templating: Femoral template is kept centered along long axis of shaft and moved vertically till center of femoral head template lies at same vertical level of planned acetabular center of rotation. If both centers coincide then this should be considered as reference point for reconstruction. If femoral template center lies medial, increase in offset should be anticipated. Excessive increase in offset should be avoided. If femoral template center lies lateral, decrease in offset is indicated and is unacceptable. Two to three millimeter circumferential cement mantle should be maintained for cemented prosthesis. Proximal fit in proximally coated and distal fit in extensively coated stem over several centimeters determines size of uncemented stem. Neck cut should be high (1–2 cm from lesser trochanter). However lower neck cut is planned with longer neck prosthesis if needs increased offset (as in case femoral head center lies lateral to planned acetabular center of rotation or protrusio).

CT scan with 3D reconstruction will give additional information regarding medial wall defect and quantification of bony defect in case of superomedial migration, so as to anticipate need of allograft as well as acetabular reconstruction cages or meshes if required.[23]

Autologous blood transfusion: Autologous blood donation can be done and stored for intraoperative transfusion if required. It can be considered specifically in bilateral simultaneous hip arthroplasty.[24] Prerequisites being predonation hemoglobin level should be > 11 gm%, weight > 25 kg, without major cardiac conditions and donation should be done at least 4 weeks prior to surgery.[25,26] Predonation of erythropoietin is also beneficial along with iron supplements to improve hemoglobin content.[5] Anemic patients with anticipated major blood loss can be considered for intraoperative blood salvage techniques.[24] Intraoperative blood salvage technique with reinfusion (autotransfusion) reduces need of homologous blood to 28%.[9] Hence autologous predonation or intraoperative blood salvage technique and reinfusion should be considered whenever indicated keeping comorbid conditions in mind.

Prerequisite for simultaneous bilateral hip arthroplasty in single anesthesia:
- Age less than 70 years
- No other comorbidities
- ASA Grade I and II
- Experienced surgeon > 25 arthroplasties/year.[27]

Operating room: Operating room should meet following standards to minimize infection especially in cases of rheumatoid arthritis, which has propensity towards it due to reduced immunity. Operating room should have positive pressure ventilation with respect to corridors and outside. Vertical laminar air flow with exhaust near floor reduces infection rate significantly.[28] HEPA filters with at least 15 to 20 air changes/hour is desirable.[29] The number of persons inside the theater should be the minimum required and number of door openings should be limited. Along with all these battery powered body exhaust suits are advisable in joint replacement surgeries.[30,31]

SURGICAL STEPS

Approach

Several approaches are described for total hip arthroplasty, however those indicated in rheumatoid arthritis taking special/difficult conditions into consideration are described. Certain precautions should be taken while exposure and dislocation in rheumatoid or say any other inflammatory arthritis in view of osteoporosis; don't put sharp retractors harshly over greater trochanter to avoid fragmentation and don't rotate femur unless femoral head is dislocated otherwise it may result in spiral fracture of shaft femur.

Posterolateral Approach

Most preferred approach adapted by surgeons for total hip arthroplasty. However, it is preferable specifically in cases that may require trochanteric osteotomy in view of difficult exposure or dislocation of femoral head, such as ankylosis, protrusion, extensive heterotropic ossification and acetabular reconstruction requiring cages and grafts.

Take 10 to 15 cms posteriorly curved incision centered 2 cm distal to tip of greater trochanter. Divide the fascia lata and gluteus maximus fascia in line of skin incision and split gluteus maximus fibers. Excision of trochanteric bursa followed by gluteus medius retraction with spike (avoid harsh retraction over greater trochanter with sharp spikes in view of osteoporosis, better don't put retractors directly over the trochanter). Detach the posterior capsule and external rotators from crest of trochanter in single layer. Incise capsule from acetabulum proximal to the piriformis and extending distally up to the capsular insertion on the proximal femur. Release of quadratus femoris subperiosteally to visualize lesser trochanter.

Trochanteric Osteotomy

Indicated in cases with anticipated difficult exposure and dislocation of femoral head, viz. protrusio and ankylosis. However, it should be avoided in severe osteolysis of greater trochanter. Standard posterolateral approach centered over greater trochanter is taken. Retraction of gluteus medius with Hohman retractor as described above with external rotator release from their insertion. Subperiosteal elevation of vastus lateralis is to be done up to 5 cms from vastus ridge. Osteotomise greater trochanter with oscillating or Gigli saw.

Posterolateral Approach with *in situ* Neck Osteotomy (Before Femoral Head Dislocation)

Neck cut fascilitates accessibility to femoral head and acetabulum. Femoral head can be removed either *en bloc* or piecemeal directly under vision. This is preferred approach by most of surgeons including senior author in protrusion and ankylosis.

Minimally Invasive Surgery

Minimally invasive surgery (MIS) can be done in uncomplicated cases provided surgeon should be experienced in performing MIS. However, it should be avoided in difficult cases of rheumatoid arthritis with anticipated difficult exposure and dislocation of femoral head, such as protrusio acetabuli and ankylosis of hip.[32]

Dislocation of Femoral Head

Dislocation of femoral head is technically demanding step requires surgeon's expertise and patience in addition to adequate surgical exposure. Also remember one should not rotate femur unless it is disengaged from acetabulum to prevent spiral fracture. Complete capsulotomy preserving anterior capsule along with marginal osteophytectomy is a prerequisite.[33] Flexion-extension at hip with adduction should be done repetitively to overcome vacuum effect at hip joint. Maximal adduction in hip flexion should bring femoral head out of acetabulum posteriorly. Also head can be levered with gouge while the maneuver to facilitate dislocation.[33] Once head is disengaged internal rotation brings head completely out of acetabulum for neck osteotomy.

Dislocation of femoral head and mobilization of femur is extremely difficult in protrusion and ankylosis. *In situ* femoral neck osteotomy should be done to mobilize femur in these cases.[34,35] Femoral head can be removed either *en bloc* or piecemeal under vision from protrusio following neck cut and mobilization of femur. Neck osteotomy in ankylosis should not be done very close to acetabulum to avoid iatrogenic fractures.

Acetabulum Preparation

Adequate acetabulum exposure should be done prior to acetabular preparation for implantation. It is done with anterior retractor placed just beneath anterior capsule, inferiorly retractor is placed just inferior to posterior 1/3 of transverse acetabular ligament. Gluteus medius and minimus are to be retracted superiorly by Steinmann pin placed 2 cm superior to superior margin of acetabulum.

Chondrolytic type of acetabulum: Acetabular reaming is to be done with sequential reamers till cancellous bleeding is seen with due attention to preservation of cancellous bed medially. Anchoring drill holes can be made superomedially for cemented prosthesis. Component 2 mm more in diameter should be introduced in case of uncemented arthroplasty.

Long-term study of cemented acetabular component: Lehtimaki et al. has shown 75% overall survival rate of cemented total hip arthroplasty in rheumatoid arthritis for mean follow-up duration of 20 years. Acetabular component survival at 10 and 15 years were 93.6 and 87% respectively in this study.[36] Other studies have shown similar survivorships of cemented hip arthroplasty in RA (75-80% survival at 20 years).[37,38] Creighton et al. found 97% survival rate (femur and acetabulum) in 10 year follow-up duration in rheumatoid arthritis. In this study 50% were having protrusio.[39] Similar results with cemented total hip arthroplasty in rheumatoid arthritis were shown in many studies for medium-term follow- up duration.[40,41] However significantly higher rate of cemented acetabular component loosening has been documented in young patients with rheumatoid arthritis and juvenile rheumatoid arthritis (20-30% revision rate).[36,39,42–46] Some have shown satisfactory results of cemented arthroplasty in young female patients with lower body weight and activity level.[42] Decreased survival rate has been reported for cemented acetabular components in rheumatoid patients with amyloidosis.[36]

Long-term study of uncemented acetabular component: Thomason et al. reported 97% survival rate of uncemented acetabular component in RA for mean follow-up duration of 7.4 years and recommends uncemented cup in all patients with rheumatoid arthritis.[47] Similar results were shown with porous coated acetabular components in rheumatoid patients.[41] Garcia Araujo et al. has reported better medium-term results of hydroxyapatite coated hip prosthesis (femoral and acetabular) in rheumatoid arthritis even in presence of osteopenia.[48]

Protrusio Acetabuli

Femoral head migrates superomedially in protrusio secondary to rheumatoid arthritis.[47] Also acetabulum is barrel-shaped with narrow opening and wide base in protrusio 2° to rheumatoid arthritis. Sciatic nerve lies close to greater trochanter in protrusion as well as ankylosis and hence prone towards injury while exposure. Intraoperatively try to keep hip in extension with knee flexion in order to avoid stretching of nerve.

Aim is restoration of center of rotation by shifting the acetabular component laterally, preserving strong medial support, medial buttressing of component with bone graft as well as cages if required and peripheral fit component placement.

Peripheral reaming should be done with expanding reamers rather than medial reaming.[49] Avoid medial reaming and try to preserve medial bone stock if any. Carefully scrape fibrocartilage from floor of acetabulum to expose bleeding cancellous bone and avoid medial wall fractures. Drill holes are to be made in periphery, i.e. ilium and ischium. Avoid drill holes in medial wall and superiorly. Grade II and III protrusio requires cancellous impaction bone graft for reconstruction.[14,15,18,22] Cancellous bone disks or slivers acquired from resected femoral head are desirable as wafers/disk conforms the irregular shape of acetabulum, also it remains adherent together on cement pressurization.[18] In addition to cancellous bone graft acetabular cages, meshes are required for reconstruction in case of bony defect in medial wall or if medial wall of acetabulum is found to be membranous intraoperatively.[50] Ranawat et al. recommends acetabular reconstruction device such as cages/mesh along with cancellous impaction grafting for severe superomedial protrusion (axial and superior migration > 1 cm).[22]

Long-term results of cemented cup in protrusio: Remodeling of acetabulum without progression of protrusio has been documented in cemented total hip arthroplasty with bone grafting done for varying grades of protrusio in rheumatoid arthritis.[18] Various authors has documented similar results with 76 to 86% survival rate of cemented total hip arthroplasty with impaction bone grafting.[22,51–53] However Clohisy and Harris documented 33% failure rate of cemented cups in protrusio in 9 to 12 years follow-up with no revisions of uncemented cup done for protrusio acetabuli. Though the medium-term results of cemented cup were good, long-term results need consideration in view of higher failure rates.[38] Specially higher failure rates were seen in cemented acetabular prosthesis for protrusio done in younger patients aged less than 50 years.[43]

Results of uncemented acetabular cup in protrusio: Acetabular remodeling with equatorial fit uncemented cup has better results according Campos et al.[16] Also Mullaji et al. reported excellent medium-term results of uncemented acetabular prosthesis with impaction bone grafting showing 100% graft consolidation with no progression of protrusio.[49] Berger reported no radiographic loosening during 7 to 11 years follow-up of uncemented acetabular reconstruction in younger patients aged less than 50 years.[54]

Ankylosis

Bony landmark of acetabulum may be obscured in case of long-standing ankylosis especially in bony ankylosis. Intraoperative status of abductors is an important factor for prediction of postoperative functional outcome. Intraoperative perception of contractions of gluteus medius and minimus can be taken as positive predictor of better functional outcome. Inferior margin of acetabulum can be marked with reference to obturator foramen. Reaming of acetabulum is to be done over the osteotomy cautiously with above mentioned reference landmark. Rest of the procedure is done similar to 1° arthroplasty preserving medial bone stock.

Results of total hip arthroplasty: The results of total hip arthroplasty in ankylosis due to rheumatoid arthritis were not been very well documented. However, literature regarding THR in spontaneous ankylosis of hip suggest good short-term results but inferior results in long-term. Various authors reported 95 to 100% survival rate for THA in spontaneous ankylosis for 10 years follow-up.[55–57] Functional improvement has also been reported post THR in ankylosis.[56,57] Kilgus et al. has shown higher failure rates of THA for ankylosis of hip done in patients less than 45 years of age.[58]

Femoral Canal Preparation

Certain precautions need to be taken while femoral canal preparation and implantation to prevent complications. Sharp retractors should not be placed directly over greater trochanter to avoid fracture owing to osteoporosis. Avoid devascularization or extensive dissection of gluteal musculature especially in ankylosed hips. Neck cut is to be taken according to preoperative planning, i.e. 1 to 2 cms from lesser trochanter. Ensure anteversion of femoral prosthesis by taking box cut in desired version. Sequential broaching is to be done as per the inventory selected. Fixation of femoral prosthesis can be chosen as per type of canal: uncemented femoral stem in type A canal, cemented femoral prosthesis must be preferred in type C canal whereas either of the two in type B femoral canal.[21] Customized narrow stem should be made available if anticipated preoperatively especially in juvenile rheumatoid patients. Restoration of vertical and horizontal offset should be checked with appropriate trial prosthesis before final implantation.

Results of Cemented Femoral Prosthesis in RA

Several authors' notified 92 to 97% survival of cemented femoral prosthesis in rheumatoid patients for mean follow-up of 10 years and up to 89% for 15 years.[36,39,42,47] However Lehtimaki and H Kautiainen noticed decreased survival rate of cemented femoral stems in males.[36] Hozack et al. reported higher failure rates of cemented femoral prosthesis in male patients with rheumatoid arthritis.[59]

Results of Uncemented Femoral Prosthesis

Though long-term results of first generation uncemented femoral stems were inferior, authors have reported satisfactory results with newer uncemented prosthesis.[47] Jana et al. reported 98% survival rate of porous coated uncemented femoral prosthesis for mean follow-up of 11 years, provided excellent surface contact is obtained with endosteal cortical bone.[41] Carlos Garcia et al. has shown excellent medium term results of hydroxyapatite coated femoral stems clinically with no radiological loosening even in relative and absolute osteopenia in a multicentric trial.[48] In a recent study of hydroxyapatite coated CAD-CAM femoral component in young patients with inflammatory polyarthropathy McCullough et al. has shown excellent medium to long-term results in skeletally mature adults with overall failure rate of 9.5% over 10 years follow-up duration.[60]

Postoperative Course and DVT Prophylaxis

Prophylactic antibiotics are given perioperatively starting from the night before surgery. The ankle pumps and static squads should start as soon as in recovery room. Patients should be trained and encouraged to do incentive spirometry along with physiotherapy specifically in bilateral arthroplasty. Graduated compression stockings, pneumatic compression devices and LMW heparins are used for DVT prophylaxis.

Postoperative Physiotherapy and Rehabilitation[10]

The aim of rehabilitation is to restore function with the intent to increase and maintain the muscle strength as well as range of motion of a joint. The balance between rest and exercise is the key to successful physiotherapy and rehabilitation in rheumatoid as well as other inflammatory polyarthropathies. It starts from preoperative period with evaluation of gait, muscle strength, range of motion of a particular joint and continues postoperatively. Postoperative rehabilitation depends on preoperative status as well as intraoperative course including the surgical approach.

Extremes of hip flexion, adduction, and internal rotation must be avoided in case of posterior/posterolateral approach has been taken, vice versa

in anterolateral approach. Weight-bearing must be protected in case of trochanteric osteotomy. Toe touch weight-bearing and active abduction must be avoided for 6 to 12 weeks postsurgery or until the osteotomy is well united. Abductor and extensor strengthening exercises should be encouraged and emphasized specially in THA done for ankylosis. Range of motion exercises should also be taught along with the strengthening exercises. Cane/crutches/walkers should be used until abductor weakness is resolved. Training regarding transfer from bed to standing position as well as toilet transfers should be taught to avoid dislocating positions. Instructions should be given to patients regarding activities of daily living in order to adapt arthroplasty lifestyle so as to prevent dislocating positions and for long-term successful outcome. In case patient wants to carry weight he/she should be instructed to carry it on the side of hip arthroplasty done.

COMPLICATIONS

Complications of arthroplasty are common in rheumatoid as well as other inflammatory arthropathies owing to immunosuppresion with DMARDs, osteoporosis, complex acetabular configurations, etc. Malchau reported five times higher revision rate in young female patients with rheumatoid arthritis.[61]

Intraoperative Complications

Sciatic nerve palsy (1-3%) is mostly neuropraxia due to traction injury. There are more chances of neural injury in protrusio and long-standing ankylosis while exposure owing to proximity towards greater trochanter. Hip should be kept in extension with knee flexion to avoid this. Intraoperative nerve conduction studies or rarely neurolysis is advisable.

Iatrogenic Fractures

Fragmentation of greater trochanter due to harsh retraction with sharp retractors directly over trochanter. This should be avoided. Spiral fracture of shaft femur can occur while dislocation due to rotational maneuvers prior to disengagement of femoral head.

Perforation of cortex can occur while broaching or uncemented femoral prosthesis implantation. It can also happen in case of previous surgery with internal fixation or juvenile rheumatoid arthritis with femur hypoplasia.[62] Similarly acetabular fractures may take place during either impaction grafting or peripheral fit uncemented implant placement.

Early Postoperative Complications

Infection: Early infection occurs in 6 months of surgery. Several authors have reported higher infection rate of arthroplasty in rheumatoid as compared to degenerative arthritis and other diagnosis.[63] It has been shown in literature that infection in rheumatoid is 1.5 to 3 times higher than osteoarthritis;[63,64] 1 to 3.7% infection rate has been reported by different authors.[63–65] Tumor necrosis factor α blockers (TNF-α) therapy in perioperative duration is associated with very high infection rate (12.5%) where as with DMARDs the infection rate is within the reported range (2%).[66] The most common organism isolated from infected arthroplasty is *Staphylococcus aureus.*[63]

Dislocation can occur most commonly in initial few weeks of postoperative period 0.7 to 3% dislocation has been reported in literature.[62,64] Patient noncompliance majorly contributes to dislocation. Also in rheumatoid it can be the resultant of excessive retroversion of femoral prosthesis, which may be secondary to valgus external rotation deformity at knee resulting in false judgment of femoral anteversion on table.[65] Rheumatoid patients have decreased tendency of healing and thus compromised capsular healing should be anticipated after dislocation. Thus abduction pillow or brace should be strictly used till at least 6 weeks postreduction.

Deep vein thrombosis and pulmonary embolism: Though subclinical deep vein thrombosis can be present in higher proportion of patients undergoing hip arthroplasty irrespective of the diagnosis, clinically significant DVT has been reported 1 to 3% in various follow-up studies.[62,18] Fatal pulmonary embolism has been reported in 1 to 3% patients not receiving any prophylaxis. Similar to infection there are very high chances of DVT in patients receiving TNF-α blockers therapy perioperatively (51%) as compared to DMARDs (26%).[66] Incidence of DVT has been reported to be low with spinal anesthesia (13%) as compared to general anesthesia (27%).[67] Fat embolism higher chances of fat embolism in simultaneous bilateral hip arthroplasty in single anesthesia.

Late Complications of Total Hip Arthroplasty in Rheumatoid Arthritis

Infection: late infection is mostly hematogenous in nature. One to two percent deep infection rate has been noticed.[36] Colville et al. suggests antibiotics should be given to patients every time infection occurs at any site to prevent bacteremia as rheumatoid hip are more susceptible to hematogenous seeding.[62] Very high infection rate are being reported in revision hip arthroplasty done for infected primary in rheumatoid arthroplasty.

Higher rate of loosening, osteolysis and subsequent failure is seen with cemented acetabular cup in younger patients with rheumatoid arthritis as well as those having amyloidosis (Table 2). Uncemented femoral prosthesis has higher failure rates in juvenile rheumatoid arthritis (JRA) patients and other inflammatory arthropathies with age less than 16 years at time of arthroplasty.

Heterotropic ossification: Two to fourteen percent symptomatic heterotropic ossification has been reported, though asymptomatic incidence being high.[62,64] Patients with rheumatoid arthritis have lesser tendency towards heterotropic ossification as compared to degenerative arthritis and ankylosing spondylitis.

Trochanteric nonunion: Trochanteric nonunion is seen in 19 to 24% cases with greater tendency of avulsion in protrusio.[18,22,62]

Periprosthetic fractures: Periprosthetic fractures are common in patients with rheumatoid arthritis owing to osteoporosis. They can be managed as per Vancouver classification system, i.e. fixation if implant is not loosened, whereas revision in

Table 2: Osteolysis and loosening of prosthesis

Author	Osteolysis and loosening femoral complication		Osteolysis and loosening acetabular complication		Follow-up in years	Remarks
	Cemented	Uncemented	Cemented	Uncemented		
McCullough JBJS 2006		9.5% HA coated			10	28.5% failure risk for JRA < 16 years
Clayton JOA 2001	7%	30%		3%	7.4	UC acetabular comp higher success in RA
AK Jana JBJS 2001		7%	54%	6%	11	
Creighton JBJS 1998	15%		16%		10	

Author	Osteolysis and loosening femoral complication	Osteolysis and loosening acetabular complication	Follow-up in years	Remarks
	Cemented	Cemented		
Chmell JBJS 1997	28%	35%	11	JRA
Severt CORR 1991	13%	13%	7.4	↑ Failure rate of cemented acetabular complications in younger patients
Unger JOA 1987		8.4%	10	
Lachiewicz JBJS 1986	8%	26%	11	JRA

case of unstable implant. Also along with all these bone mineral density should be improved with antiresorptive therapy alone or in combination.

Author's Experiences and Recommendations

The senior author has significant experience in handling arthroplasty for rheumatoid arthritis and takes the opportunity to share his experiences regarding the same. We have seen patients in various stages of the rheumatoid and the epidemiology seems to be consistent with the literature worldwide. We have also treated rheumatoid patients with crippling deformities at hip and encountered poor perineal hygiene as a consistent finding in these patients along with the whole consortium of rheumatoid sequelae.

It poses additional difficulty in view of proximity to the surgical site and difficultly in adductor tenotomy. We encountered many difficult situations as mentioned above with majority being osteoporosis. We have experience of simultaneous hip and knee arthroplasties in patients with rheumatoid arthritis (Table 3). We had opportunity to replace all four joints in four patients and ipsilateral hip and knee in twelve patients. The senior author personally feels it is better to operate hip followed by ipsilateral knee in single stage due to positional difficulties in case of bilateral hip and knee involvement. We had shown to perform bilateral arthroplasty in single anesthesia provided patients is ASA grade I or II, age less than 70 years and no comorbidities. We prefer spinal and epidural combined anesthesia as there are fewer chances of deep vein thrombosis and other complications. Also better postoperative analgesia can be achieved with epidural infusion postoperatively which aids in successful physiotherapy. We recommend keeping the epidural catheter *in situ* for the second stage which is planned within a week keeping difficult anesthesia into consideration, provided general and medical condition of patient permits. DMARDs should be considered as per recommendations; however we propose to avoid TNF-α blockers perioperatively. Strict antibiotic protocol and asepsis is followed perioperatively. Posterolateral approach is usually preferred with generous incision. Gluteus maximus tendon release is required mostly in these cases along with extensive capsular release. Hip extension and knee flexion is must to avoid sciatic nerve injury. Also circumferentially defining femoral neck before *in situ* osteotomy in protrusion and ankylosis is must. We strongly recommend anterior capsular release and prefer position of hip in flexion while placing anterior retractors and reaming to avoid possibility of injury to anterior neurovascular structures. In cases of ankylosis, we start reaming over the neck followed by head extending up to medial wall of acetabulum with the properly placed anterior retractor. In juvenile rheumatoid arthritis stunted growth is usual phenomenon and hence hypoplasia should be anticipated and customized narrow femoral stems and acetabular cups should be made available on the day of surgery. Uncemented hydroxyapatite coated cups can be used in all patients. While cemented acetabular implant in rheumatoid can be preferred in older patients, young females with low activity levels and lower body weight. Cancellous bone slivers are required in grade II and III protrusio for reconstruction. Antiprotrusio cages are indicated in addition to cancellous bone graft for grade III protrusio, medial wall defect, membranous medial wall found intraoperatively and superomedial migration of femoral head more

Table 3: Author's recommendations for total hip arthroplasty in rheumatoid arthritis

Acetabulum prosthesis	Patient type and acetabular configuration	Remarks
Cemented	Older age Young female – low body weight and activity	Anchoring holes in ilium and ischium only Avoid drilling medial wall
Uncemented	All age group (even in osteopenia) Protrusio Gr I	
Uncemented and BG	Protrusio Gr II	Protrusio: Peripheral rim fit Lateralize cup and restore anatomic center of rotation
Antiprotrusio cages/meshes and bone graft	Protrusio Gr III Medial wall defect Membranous medial wall Superomedial migration of femoral head > 1 cm	

Femoral prosthesis	Type of canal (Dossick)	Remarks
Cemented	A and B	Customised narrow prosthesis in JRA
Uncemented	C and B	High failure in JRA < 16 years Careful while broaching and implantation

...han 1 cm. Hydroxyapatite coated femoral prosthesis is preferred in Dossick type A canal where as cemented prosthesis in type C canal. Author prefers pneumatic compression device and TED stockings postoperatively. Ankle pumps and static quads should be started as soon as possible. Abductor and extensor strengthening should be emphasized especially in conversion total hip arthroplasty in case of ankylosis. The patients are mobilized as soon as possible, mostly on 2nd postoperative day. Assisted ambulation with walker is preferred initially for few days and for longer duration in conversion hip arthroplasty till adequate abductor and extensor strength is regained. Patients are given adequate postural training, gait training as well as transfer training postoperatively, and can be discharged after satisfactory stair climbing. DMARDs should be readjusted once wound heals according to rheumatologist recommendations. Also osteoporosis should be taken care with appropriate drug regimen. The hip arthroplasty in patients with rheumatoid arthritis is a complex procedure which necessitates surgical expertise. However, the treatment is incomplete without overall patient care in the continuum of disease.

REFERENCES

1. Storey GD. Heberden Historical series: Alfred Baring Garrod (1819–1907). Rheumatology 2001;40:1189-90.
2. Sherine E Gabriel, Kaleb Michaud. Epidemiological studies in incidence, prevalence, mortality, and comorbidity of the rheumatic diseases. Arthritis Research and Therapy 2009;11:229.
3. Lehtimaki MY, Kaarela K, Hamalainen MMJ. Incidence of Hip Involvement and Need for Total Hip Replacement in Rheumatoid Arthritis: An Eight-year Follow-up Study Scandinavian. Journal of Rheumatology 1986;15(4):387-91.
4. Lipsky PE. Rheumatoid arthritis chapter 312 in Harrisons Principles of Internal medicine 15th edition. E Braunwarld et al. (Eds) USA: McGraw Hill publication 2001. pp.1928-37.
5. Mylene V Matti, Nigel E Sharrock. Anesthesia on the Rheumatoid Patients. Rheumatic Diseases Clin North Am 1998;24(1):19.
6. Ronald MacKenzie C, Nigel E Sharrock. Perioperative medical consideration in patients with rheumatoid arthritis. Rheumatic Diseases Clin of North Am 1998;24(1).
7. Robert P Dunbar, Michael M Alexiades: Decision making in rheumatoid arthritis: Determining Surgical Priorities. Rheumatic Diseases Clinics of North America 1998;24(1):35-54.
8. Solomon DH, Goodson NJ, Katz JN, Weinblatt ME, Avorn J, Setoguchi S, Canning C, Schneeweiss S. Patterns of cardiovascular risk in rheumatoid arthritis Ann Rheum Dis 2006;65:1608-12.
9. Endresen GKM, Spiechowicz J, Pahle JA, Espeland B. Intraoperative Autotransfusion in Reconstructive Hip Joint Surgery of Patients with Rheumatoid Arthritis and Ankylosing Spondylitis. Scandinavian Journal of Rheumatology 1991;20(1):28-35.
10. Sandy B Ganz, Louis L Harris. Trends in orthopedic surgery for rheumatoid arthritis: general overview of rehabilitation in the rheumatoid patient. Rheumatic Diseases Clinics of North America 1998;24(1):181.
11. Herwig Pieringer, Ulrike Stuby, George Biesenbach. Patients with rheumatoid arthritis undergoing surgery: how should we deal with antirheumatic treatment? Semin Arthritis Rheum 2007;36:278-86.
12. Eggli S, Pisan M, Muller ME. The value of preoperative planning for total hip arthroplasty. J Bone Joint Surg [Br] 1998;80(B):382-90.
13. McElwain JP, Sheehan JM. Bilateral hip and knee replacement for rheumatoid arthritis J Bone Joint Surg Br 1985;67-B(2):261-5.
14. Ranawat and Zahn MG. Role of bone grafting in correction of protrusion acetabuli by total hip arthroplasty. JOA 1986;1:131-7.
15. Colin CR Dunlop, Charles Wynn Jones, Nicola Maffulli. Protrusio Acetabuli Bulletin, Hospital for Joint Diseases 2005;62(3 and 4):105-14.
16. Campos JPE, Schwartsmann CR, Faria M, Bernabé AC, Gomes M, Luca Junior G. Otto pelvis remodeling after total hip arthroplasty. Acta Ortop Bras 2009;17(1):58-61.
17. Sotelo-Garza A, Charnley J. The results of Charnley arthroplasty of the hip performed for protrusio acetabuli. Clin Orthop 1978;132:12-8.
18. Philip Hirst, Max Esser, John CM Murphy, Kevin Hardinge. Bone grafting for protrusio acetabuli during total hip replacement. A review of the Wrightington method in 61 hips. J Bone Joint Surg Br 1987;69-B(2):229-33.
19. Armbuster TG, Guerra J, Resnick D, et al. The adult hip: an anatomic study. Radiology 1978;128:1-10.

20. Gates HS, Poletti SC, Callaghan JJ, McCollum DE. Radiographic measurements in protrusio acetabuli. J Arthroplasty 1989;4:347-51.
21. Dossick PH, Dorr LD, Gruen T, Saberi MT. Techniques for preoperative planning and postoperative evaluation of noncemented hip arthroplasty. Tech Orthop 1991;6(3):1-6.
22. Ranawat CS, Dorr LD and Inglis AE. Total hip arthroplasty in protrusio acetabuli of rheumatoid arthritis. J Bone Joint Surg Am 1980;62:1059-65.
23. Barmeira E, Dubowitza B, Roffmana M. Computed tomography in the assessment and planning of complicated total hip replacement. Acta Orthopaedica 1982;53(4):597-604.
24. Mark Tenholder, Fred D Cushner. Intraoperative blood management in joint replacement surgery Orthopedics 2004;27(6):S663.
25. Brian G Feagan, Cindy J Wong, William C Johnston, Ramiro Arellano, Nigel Colterjohn, Keyvan Karkouti Transfusion practices for elective orthopedic surgery Canadian Medical Association Journal 2002;166(3):310-4.
26. Elizabeth S Vanderlinde, Joanna M Heal, Neil Blumberg. Autologous transfusion. British Medical Journal 2002;324:772-5.
27. Gary J Hooper, Nikki M Hooper, Alastair G Rothwell, Toni Hobbs. Bilateral total joint arthroplasty: the early results from the New Zealand National Joint Registry. J Arthroplasty 2009;24(8):1174-7.
28. Mangram AJ. Hospital Infection Control Practices Advisory Committee (HICPAC) and Centers for Disease Control and Prevention (CDC): guidelines for prevention of surgical site infection. Infect Control Hosp Epidemiol 1999;24(4):247-78.
29. Campbells. Operative orthopedic. S Terry Canale (Ed), Tenth edition Mosby 2003;1:238.
30. Whyte W, Lidwell OM, Lowbury EJL, Blowers R. Suggested bacteriological standards for air in ultraclean operating theaters. Journal of Hospital Infection 1983;42:133-9.
31. Torbjorn A, Dalen N, Jorbeck H, Hoborn J. Air contamination during hip and knee arthroplasties: horizontal laminar flow vs conventional ventilation. Acta Orthopaedica Scandinavia 1995;66(1):17-20.
32. Chitranjan S Ranawat, Amar S Ranawat. Minimally invasive total joint arthroplasty: where are we going? J bone Joint Surg Am 2003;85:2070-1.
33. Eftekhar N. Indications and contraindications for total hip replacement; Chapter 8 in Principles of Total Hip Arthroplasty. N Eftekhar (Ed). Saint Louis: Mosby 1978.p.207.
34. Bhende H. Total Hip Replacement following acetabular fractures. Indian Journal of Orthopaedics 2002;36(1):33-5.
35. Barrett S Brown, Michael H Huo. Conversion Total Hip Replacement in the Adult Hip. John J Callaghan Aaron G Rosenberg, et al. (Eds), 2nd, Lippincot Williams and Wilkins 2007; chapter 107.
36. Lehtimaki MY, Kautiainen H, Lehto MUK, Hamalainen MMJ. Charnley Low Friction Arthroplasty in Rheumatoid Patients. A survival study up to 20 years. Journal of Arthroplasty 1999;14(6):657-61.
37. Joshi AB, Porter ML, Trail IA. Long-term results of Charnley Low Friction Arthroplasty in young patients. J Bone Joint Surg Br 1993;75:616.
38. Schulte KR, Callaghan JJ, Kelley SS, Johnston RC. The outcome of Charnley total hip arthroplasty with cement after a minimum twenty-year follow-up: the result of one surgeon. J Bone Joint Surg Am 1993;75:961.
39. Mark G Creighton, Olenjniczak JP, Richard C Johnston. Total hip arthroplasty with cement in patients who have rheumatoid arthritis. A minimum ten-year follow-up study. J Bone Joint Surg Am 1998;80:1439-46.
40. Unger AS, Inglis AE, Ranawat CS, Johanson NA. Total hip arthroplasty in rheumatoid arthritis. A long-term follow-up study. Journal of Arthroplasty 1987;2:191-7.
41. Jana AK, Engh CA Jr, Lewandowski PJ, Hopper RH Jr, Engh CA. Total hip arthroplasty using porous coated femoral components in patients with rheumatoid arthritis. J Bone Joint Surg Br 2001;83(B):686-90.
42. Lachiewicz PF, McCaskill B, Inglis A, Ranawat CS, Rosenstein BD. Total hip arthroplasty in juvenile rheumatoid arthritis. Two-eleven year results. J Bone Joint Surg Am 1986;68:502-8.
43. Ballard WT, Callaghan JJ, Sullivan PM, Johnston RC. The results of improved cementing techniques for total hip arthroplasty in patients less than fifty years old. A ten years follow-up study. J Bone Joint Surg Am 1994;76-A:959-64.
44. Sarmiento A, Ebramzadeh E, Gogan WJ, Mckellop. Total hip arthroplasty with cement. A long-term radiographic analysis in patients older than fifty and younger than fifty years. J Bone Joint Surg Am 1990;72(A):1470-6.
45. Severt R, Wood R, Cracchiolo A, Amstutz HC. Longterm follow-up of cemented total hip arthroplasty in rheumatoid arthritis. Clin Orthop 1991;265:137-45.

46. Chmell MJ, Scott RG, Thomas WH, Sledge MD. Total hip arthroplasty with cement for juvenile rheumatoid arthritis. J Bone Joint Surg Am 1997;79:44.

47. H Clayton Thomason III, Paul F Lachiewicz. The influence of technique on fixation of primary total hip arthroplasty in patients with rheumatoid arthritis. J of Arthroplasty 2001;16(5):628-34.

48. Carlos Garcia Araujo, Julian Fernandez, Alphons Tonino. Rheumatoid arthritis and hydroxyapatite-coated hip prostheses. Journal of Arthroplasty 1998; 13(6):660-7.

49. Arun B Mullaji, Satyajit V Marawar. Primary total hip arthroplasty in protrusio acetabuli using impacted morsellized bone grafting and cementless cups. A medium-term radiographic review. Journal of Arthroplasty 2007;22(8):1143-9.

50. Donald E McCollum, James A Nunley, John L Harrelson. Bone grafting in total hip replacement for acetabular protrusion. J Bone Joint Surg Am 1980; 62-A(7):1065.

51. Welten ML, Schreurs BW, Buma P, et al. Acetabular-reconstruction with impacted morsellized cancellous bone autograft and cemented primary total hiparthroplasty: a 10 to 17-year follow-up study. J Arthroplasty 2000;15:819.

52. Rosenberg AWJ, Schreurs WB, et al. Impacted morsellized bone grafting and cemented primary total hip arthroplasty for acetabular protrusion in patients with rheumatoid arthritis. Acta Orthop Scand 2000;71:143.

53. Schreurs BW, Slooff TJ, et al. Acetabular reconstruction with bone impaction grafting and a cemented-cup. Clin Orthop 2001;393:202.

54. Berger RA, Jacobs JJ, et al. Primary cementless acetabular reconstruction in patients younger than 50 years old. Clin Orthop 1997;344:216.

55. Strathy GM, Fitzgerald RH. Total hip arthroplasty in the ankylosed hip. J Bone Joint Surg Am 1988;70:963-6.

56. Joshi AB, Markovic L, Hardinge K, et al. Conversion of a fused hip to total hip arthroplasty. J Bone Joint Surg Am 2002;84:1335-41.

57. Hamadouche M, Kerboull L, Meunier A, et al. Total hip arthroplasty for the treatment of ankylosed hips. J Bone Joint Surg Am 2001;83:992-8.

58. Kilgus DJ, Amstutz HC, Wolgin MA, et al. Joint replacement for ankylosed hips. J Bone Joint Surg Am 1990;72:45-54.

59. Hozack WJ, Rothman RH, Booth RE, et al. Survivorship analysis of 1041 Charnleys total hip arthroplasties. Journal of Arthroplasty 1990;5:41.

60. McCullough CJ, Remedios D, Tytherleigh-Strong G, Hua J, Walker PS. The use of hydroxyapatite coated CAD-CAM femoral components in adolescents and young adults with inflammatory polyarthropathy 10 year results. J Bone Joint Surg Br 2006;88(B):860-4.

61. Malchau H, Herberts P, Ahnfelt L, Johnell O. Prognosis of total hip replacement: Swedish National Hip Arthroplasty Register. Presented at the 64th annual meeting of the American Academy of orthopedic Surgeons, Atlanta, Feb 1996.

62. James Colville, Pauli Raunio. Charnley low – friction arthroplasties of the hip in rheumatoid arthritis. J Bone Joint Surg Br 1978;60-B(4):498-503.

63. Bongartz T, Halligan CS, Osmon DR, Reinalda MS, Bamlet WR, Crowson CS, et al. Incidence and risk factors of prosthetic joint infection after total hip or knee replacement in patients with rheumatoid arthritis. Arthritis and Rheumatism 2008;59(12):1713-20.

64. Chitranjan S Ranawat. Surgical management of rheumatoid hip. Rheumatic Diseases Clinics of North America 1998;24(1):129-40.

65. Poss R, Ewald FC, Thomas WH, Sledge CB. Complications of total hip arthroplasty in patients with rheumatoid arthritis. J Bone Joint Surg Am 1976;58:1130-3.

66. Kosei, Kawakami, Katsunori Ikari, Koichiro Kawamura, So Tsukahara, Takuji Iwamoto, Koichiro Yano, et al. Complications and features after joint surgery in rheumatoid arthritis patients treated with tumor necrosis factor blocker: Perioperative interruption of tumor necrosis factor blockers decrease complications? Rheumatology 2010;49: 341-7.

67. Davis FM, Laurenson VG, Gillispie WJ, Wells JE, Foate J, Newman E. Deep vein thrombosis after total hip replacement: a comparison between spinal and general anesthesia. J Bone Joint Surg Br 1989;71(B):181-5.

9 | Total Hip Arthroplasty for Old Tuberculous Hip Arthritis

Y Kharbanda

Hips affected by tuberculosis infection may lead to irreversible damage to articular surfaces with secondary arthritis or spontaneous fusion. Few of these hips may have been operated and present as Girdlestone excision. Patients with such hips are now being accepted for total hip arthroplasty (THA).

This condition is more prevalent in Asian countries where tuberculosis is still very common disease. Patients with tuberculous disease of hip present in advanced stages of disease and are referred for total hip arthroplasty. Hence total hip arthroplasty in old tuberculous arthritis has emerged a difficult problem due to following reasons:

1. Recrudescence of infection
2. Difficulties in surgical techniques.

RECRUDESCENCE OF INFECTION

It is well recognized that recrudescence of infection may occur in such joints even after they have been quiescent for many years such recrudescence of infection is a major complication and may lead to complete failure.

Reports of low friction arthroplasty in patients with tuberculous arthritis of the hip which has been quiescent are encouraging. Hardinge, Cleary and Charnley (1979) reported no infection in 27 healed tuberculous hips after a mean follow-up of 32 months. Jupiter et al. (1981) reported no infection in a series of 7 patients who were given antituberculous therapy before operation with a mean follow-up of 43 months. Kim et al. (1979) reported one case of reactivation of tuberculous infection in a series of

20 patients despite antituberculous treatment before surgery. Laforgia et al. (1988) reported only one case of recrudescence of tuberculosis in 72 arthroplasties in old tubercular hips. Kim et al. (1988) reported 3 case of reactivation of tuberculosis in 60 patients treated by Charnley low friction arthroplasty and followed for 8 to 13 years.

From all the above reports, it is clear that incidence of recrudescence is low but it can occur in a patient undergoing THA for an old tuberculous arthritis of hip.

Timing of the Operation

The length of time of apparent freedom from active infection should not be a deciding factor as to whether to operate.

Hardinge et al. recommended a long waiting period that is after sinuses had not drained for twenty years or after the hip had been ankylosed for more than ten years. This was in the era when modern tuberculosis drugs were not available and patient was treated with traditional ways of treatment. In contrast Johnson et al. emphasized that the length of time of inactive infection should not be a decisive factor and pointed out that there always is some risk of persistence or reactivation of the infection.

Kim et al. (1987) and Jupiter et al. (1981) reported a lower reactivation rate when THA was performed 10 years after the tuberculosis treatment. Today, in the era when THA is a very common operation, patient demands a more functional hip. There are a few reports where immediate THA is done for the treatment of active tuberculosis (please see section below).

Reactivation of tuberculosis can largely be prevented by appropriate antituberculosis chemotherapy and surgical treatment though some authors report recrudescence even after long periods of quiescence (Dolanc 1972, McCullough 1977, Johnson et al. 1979).

Surgery for treatment may include debridement, excision of sinuses, Girdlestone operation or arthrodesis. Most appropriate time has not been mentioned in any print literature, however, we believe that once tuberculosis infection is cured with modern antituberculosis chemotherapy (about one year), it may be appropriate to carry out THA.

When to Begin and Duration of Antituberculosis Treatment

The question as to when to begin antituberculosis chemotherapy and how long to continue it before and after the THA remains controversial. Jupiter et al. recommended that patients who have never received modern antituberculosis chemotherapy should be treated with one modern drug for at least one year before THA. Johnson et al. emphasized that prophylactic antituberculos therapy should be routinely provided in all patients, they recommended that a full dosage be administered starting immediately before operation and continuing for at least 12 to 18 months depending on serial readings of ESR. Kim et al. (1987) concluded from their study that routine prophylactic chemotherapy before THA is not necessary unless: (1) There is suspicion or evidence of an active infection, (2) The duration of the quiescent period of infection before the operation is less than ten years, or (3) If the patients had not received modern antituberculous chemotherapy continuously for at least three months before the operation.

Current Recommendations

Prophylactic chemotherapy should be continued for all patients where the duration of quiescent period of infection before the operation is less than ten years. Drug regime consisting of rifampicin and isoniazid should be started three weeks before operation and continued six months after operation. In case histology and bacteriological sampling at operation from hip joint are positive for tuberculosis, full 12 to 18 months of antituberculous chemotherapy should be given. Serial, readings of ESR may be helpful to decide the duration of postoperation chemotherapy.

Patients who have the duration of quiescent period of infection is more than ten years, prophylaxis with antituberculous chemotherapy may not be given provided there are no clinical signs of active disease and histological and bacteriological sampling from hip at joint the time of operation is negative.

Reactivation of Infection after THA

Leforgia et al. (1988) believed that all patients with previous tuberculous infection who are offered hip arthroplasty should be given a preoperative course of antituberculous drugs, unless it is known that they have already had such treatment. Johnson et al. (1979) believe that infection remains dormant for a long time and histological and bacteriological sampling at operation from hip joint may prove negative and serial readings of ESR may be of little value. These facts make a strong case for routine prophylactic antituberculous therapy in all cases. Kim et al. (1988) believe that reactivation of tuberculosis can largely be prevented by appropriate antituberculous chemotherapy. Eshola et al. (1988) recommend drug regime of rifampicin and isoniazid for three weeks before operation and six to nine months after operation. The reason for this policy is to reduce the disastrous effect of reactivation of tuberculosis.

Reactivation of Infection—Treatment Recommendation

To date there is no agreement on this question—best choice of treatment for the reactivation of infection that occurs after THA.

Johnson et al. (1979) removed the prosthesis in order to control infection. McCulhongh (1977) treated with antituberculous chemotherapy alone without removing the prosthesis. Kim et al. (1987)

treated with a combination of debridement of the sinus tract and chemotherapy. In their experience reactivation of the infection or a recurrent draining sinus can be controlled satisfactorily with chemotherapy alone or with a combination of chemotherapy and debridement of the sinus tract without removal of prosthesis.

THA in Active Tuberculosis of the Hip

Total hip arthroplasty in a hip with current tuberculosis infection is a controversial issue due to potential risk of reactivation of tuberculosis. Charnley advised against it because of high risk. Many authors have recommended a long internal between the treatment of the active infection and total hip arthroplasty.

Kim et al. (1987) and Jupiter et al. (1981) reported a lower reactivation rate when THA was performed ten years after the tuberculosis treatment.

Excision arthroplasty can be employed either as a primary or as a salvage operation. It produces a hip that is free of pain and infection, increases the range of motion, corrects the deformity, and tends to yield permanent results. These desirable features, however have to be balanced against the disadvantages of shortening of limb, an abnormal gait, instability of joint, fatigability and need of an aid for walking.

Arthrodesis is another operation used extensively in past as the procedure for the treatment of tuberculous infection of the hip joint. The rate of nonunion is between 6 to 70% and even when the operation is successful, the patients have back pain, pain in the knee and slow, asymmetrical and arrhythmic gait.

Resection arthroplasty or arthrodesis may relieve the pain and control infection, but function of the hip is unsatisfactory. Total hip arthroplasty has been well established as a successful form of treatment, but it is unclear whether THA should be performed in a patient with current infection or wait until the infection treatment is completed.

A few cases of THA in patients with active tuberculosis have been reported. Kim et al. reported successful Charnley low friction arthroplasties in patients with tuberculosis of the hip, including eight cases with active disease. Yoon et al. (2005) reported the results of primary THA in seven patients with advanced active tuberculous arthritis of the hip and had lost the chance of preserving the hip without replacement surgery. They concluded that THA in advanced active tuberculosis of the hip is a safe procedure providing symptomatic relief and functional improvement. Patients with infected sinus tracts extended into the pelvis or deep into the thigh may not be a good indication for immediate THA because the reactivation may occur if the infected tissues cannot be completely debrided. In such cases, two stage operation may be preferable. Yoon et al. (2001) reported THA in active tuberculosis in 3 cases. They concluded that the important issue is whether infected tissue can be debrided completely. They started antituberculous chemotherapy 2 weeks before the surgery and continued it for 1 year after the surgery. Yadav et al. (2009) concluded that when the infected tissue can be debrided and adequate antituberculous chemotherapy has been instituted the outcome of THA may not be adversely affected. THA in the tuberculous hip has a low-risk of reactivation and produces good functional result. Sindhu et al. (2009) concluded that THA in presence of active tuberculosis of hip is a safe procedure when preoperative chemotherapy is commenced and continued for an extended period after the operation.

We believe that more reports on long-term results are needed to perform THA in active disease. Important issues are institution of antituberculous chemotherapy preoperatively and postoperatively. It is of prime importance that at surgery infected tissue can be debrided completely. Unless the above criterion is met a safe and gold standard 2 stage procedure should be carried out.

Clinical presentation of tuberculosis arthritis may be in various forms:
• Anklylosed hips with quiescent infection
• Girdlestone—excision of head and neck
• Subluxed or dislocated hips
• Destruction of acetabalum and bone defects
• Gradually worsening arthritis.

Indications for THA may be straight forward in most of the above forms of tuberculous arthritis. The predominant symptom is pain and disability.

Pain in the hip is present when there is no ankylosis. Fibrous ankylosis, subluxation of hip and Girdlestone hip may also cause pain in the hip. Ankylosis provides a durable, painless and stable hip. However, in the long-term, especially when the hip is in a poor functional position, ankylosis of the hip can be responsible for pain and degenerative changes.

Diagnosis of tuberculosis is difficult when presentation is identical to gradually worsening arthritis. Figure 1 illustrates an example of tuberculosis of hip that presented as a gradually worsening arthritis. A 23-years-old lady presented with pain in left hip and difficulty in walking for four months. There were no constitutional symptoms of low grade temperature, loss of appetite or weight loss. Clinical examination revealed restricted range of motion in the hip joint. Blood tests were normal (ESR 15; CRP < 0.6) radiological examination revealed joint space narrowing and arthritis in the hip joint. MRI scans revealed mild effusion and there was no destruction of the head or acetabulum. CT-guided aspiration was inconclusive. Nine months later, she presented with advanced destruction of the hip (Figure 2). Excision of head and debridement was done. Histological examination confirmed tuberculosis.

SURGICAL DIFFICULTIES

Most of the literature is written about the problems of reactivation of tuberculosis infection after THA. In addition, there are scientific articles in the literature highlighting the problems of performing THA in active tuberculosis and advanced arthritis of hip. These problems are mainly focused at controversy issue due to potential risk of reactivation of tuberculosis. Not much has been written about the surgical difficulties encountered in THA for old tuberculous arthritis of hip (Figure 3). In this part of this section, these problems will be discussed. The surgical challenges encountered are as given below:

- Scarring, adhesions in the hip region
- Shortening—excessive scarring
- Anatomic distortion of acetabulum and femur
- Limb-length discrepancy.

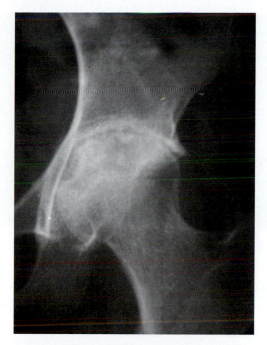

Figure 1: Tuberculosis of hip

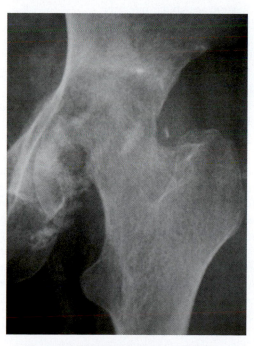

Figure 2: Advanced destruction of the hip (post-tuberculosis)

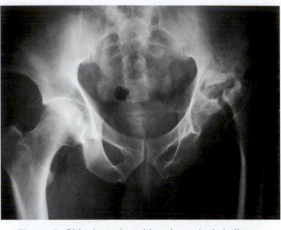

Figure 3: Old tuberculous hip—A surgical challenge

Acetabulum Reconstruction

The goals of acetabular reconstruction are to achieve a lasting functional outcome. Principles of acetabular reconstruction are:
- Restore hip mechanics and center of rotation
- Restore acetabular integrity
- Ensure acetabular component coverage
- Secure rigid graft fixation
- Secure rigid prosthesis fixation

The technical challenges in acetabular reconstruction falls under the headings of:
1. Difficult exposure such as in ankylosis and long-standing girdlestone
2. Bone defects that makes stable implant fixation difficult to achieve.

Successful acetabular reconstruction requires familiarity with potential problems and access to the tools required to deal with these problems. Careful preoperative planning is required. The surgeon must determine optimum socket placement, type of fixation—cemented or cementless, size of the component, whether bone graft is required or not and how the exposure of the acetabulum can be achieved. Best time to make these determinations is during preoperative planning.

Preoperative Planning

Preoperative assessment of acetabulum should be carried out in respect of following problems:

- Acetabular orientation
- Center of rotation
- Acetabular bone defects.

Acetabular Orientation

The orientation of the face of the acetabulum is a primary function of the bone anatomy of the pelvis and a secondary function of the peri-pelvic soft tissue. Soft tissue contracture and leg-length inequality may lead to secondary changes in acetabular orientation. The orientation of the acetabulum will change as the patient moves from the operating table to the upright position. A fixed adduction contracture will elevate the pelvis to the adducted side and flexion contracture will functionally shorten an extremity. The presence of fixed contracture of soft tissues and pelvic obliquity should be noted preoperatively and specifically managed surgically to avoid component malposition.

During operation, it is very important to identify all the walls of acetabulum by adequate exposure. These walls act as guide to position the component (Figures 4A and B). In case of bony defects, position of the patient should be taken into consideration and cup orientation determined as shown in Figure 5. The handle of the cup insertion jig should be at 45° inclination from horizontal and in 20° anteversion (Figure 5).

Center of Rotation

Placement of the acetabular component in the correct anatomic location is critical for restoration of normal biomechanics. The aim is to restore the normal lever arm for the abductor muscles of the hip as well as the normal joint reactive forces.

Method to locate correct anatomic position of acetabulum: There are various commonly used measures of hip joint position. Ranawat et al. developed a method to locate the correct anatomic position of the acetabulum in deformed hips that facilitates preoperative templating. Figure 6 is a diagram of a normal pelvis showing the placement of Ranawat's triangle.

The acetabular teardrop varies little with slight degree of pelvic obliquity and may be the most

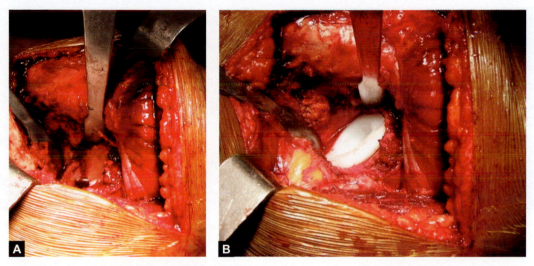

Figures 4A and B: Identification of acetabular walls and insertion of cup

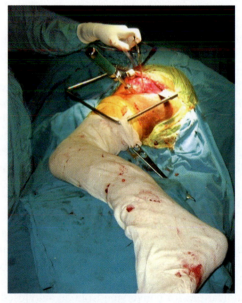

Figure 5: Position of jig for cup orientation

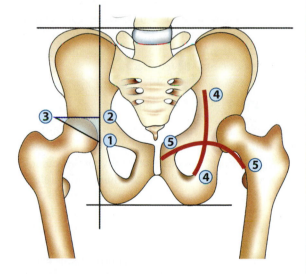

Figure 6: The method of calculating the anatomic position of the acetabulum as described by Ranawat et al. Parallel horizontal lines are drawn at the level of the ischial tuberosities and iliac crests. These lines are connected by a perpendicular line that passes through a point (1) located 5 mm medial to intersection between Shenton's line (5) and Kohler's line (4). A second point (2) is located on the perpendicular line superior to point 1, at a distance equal to one-fifth of the pelvic height measured between the two horizontal lines. From point 2, another perpendicular line is drawn laterally to point 3, which equals the distance between 1 and 2. The triangle between 1, 2 and 3 locates the acetabulum of a normal hip, with the lines 2-3 passing through the subchondral bone of the acetabulum

useful landmark. It is almost never destroyed even in advanced tuberculous arthritis (Figure 7).

Acetabular Bone Defects

Evaluation and understating of acetabular bone defects will aid in determining the best approach to

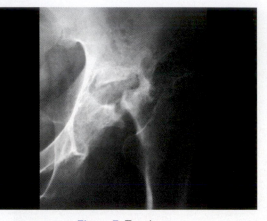

Figure 7: Teardrop

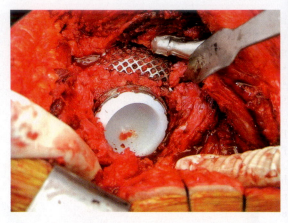

Figure 8: Acetabular bone defect superiorly—autograft and mesh used to fill the defect

the hip, whether bone graft might be required, and the appropriate equipment to have available (Figure 8).

Evaluation of anterior and posterior bone defects will require Judet views. In cases of large defects, computerized tomography with three-dimensional reconstruction may be required.

Exposure of the Acetabulum

The goals in the surgical approach to the difficult acetabulum are to see all the walls of acetabulum and bone defects, which require moving the femur to allow visualization of the acetabulum, and to release soft tissue contracture. Stiff or ankylosed hips will often require osteotomy of the femoral neck *in situ*, in order to mobilize the proximal femur sufficiently to see the acetabulum.

Acetabular cavity is filled with fibrous tissue in case of girdlestone arthroplasty. It is difficult to identify the walls of acetabulum in such cases. I have found it convenient to locate the inferior rim of acetabulum which is almost never destroyed and work my way from here to identify the other areas of acetabulum.

Capsular and ligamentous contracture are common in hips with an abnormal center of rotation, shortening and previous incisions. The longer the duration of the altered hip center or extremity shortening, the less likely it is to be correctable without complete capsulotomy and release or resection of involved musculotendenous

units. Previous surgery creates scarring that varies in severity. It is unusual to expect correction of leg-length discrepancy that exceeds one inch in the case of long-standing leg-length discrepancy. The limiting factor in lengthening is scarred and retracted abductor mechanism and sometimes sciatic nerve.

Finally, closure of these difficult hips entails appropriate tensioning of the abductor mechanism. In hips where a higher center of rotation has been accepted (long-standing Gridlestone arthroplasty) distal translation of the osteotomized trochanter is preferred in order to tension the abductor mechanism.

THA IN ANKYLOSED HIPS

It is a technical challenge for the surgeon, mainly because of difficult exposure. Abductor mechanism may be atrophic or absent making the recovery difficult.

Indications for conversion from an ankylosed hip to an arthroplasty include:
- Pain in the low back and ipsilateral knee
- Need for improved mobility
- Limb-length discrepancy.

Whereas relief of low back pain is an attainable goal, many patients will show only minimal functional improvements, with persistent limp and weakness of the hip girdle muscles (Figures 9 and 10). A successful outcome after conversion of ankylosed hip to an arthroplasty is dependent on the diagnosis or etiology of the ankylosis (whether spontaneous or surgically created)

• Indication for operation
• Length of time between fusion and arthroplasty
• Age of the patient.

The arthroplasty failure rate has been high in patients under 50 years of age with a history or previous surgery.

The technique for exposure of the ankylosed hip generally requires osteotomy of the greater trochanter for exposure of the femoral neck and acetabulum. Many authors have described exposure without osteotomy of greater trochanter. The femoral neck must be cut *in situ*. Exposure can be difficult because of distorted bony anatomy and contracture of surrounding soft tissues. Attempts at lengthening more than one inch may lead to complications (sciatic nerve injury). Amstutz and Sakal reported leg lengthening of up to 6 cm without complication and Hardinge et al. noted a maximum increase of 4 cm.

The goal in this group of patients should be to place the center of rotation of the hip in the anatomic location. The anatomic location is the most favorable with regard to joint mechanics and it places the residual abductor muscles at their greatest mechanical advantage. However, the strength of the abductor muscles postoperatively seems to be related to preoperative muscle mass as well as to the placement of the hip center.

Surgical consideration in arthrodesis of hip: If arthrodesis of the hip is present, the osteotomy should be performed as close to the acetabulum as possible. A trochanteric slide may be necessary for exposure. Following femoral neck osteotomy and shaft mobilization, the acetabular reamers should be centered around the fovea. The depth of reaming is established at the medial extent of residual foveal soft tissue by use of a depth gauge via a drill hole through the medial wall. On the femoral side, a high speed drill may be necessary to open the intramedullary canal. A long intramedullary guide rod and cannulated reamers can help establish a neutral femoral axis. It is advantageous for the femoral stem to have sufficient offset to restore abductor biomechanics and improve

range of motion. It is important to obtain intraoperative radiographs with trial components in place.

The most common complications after conversion to total hip arthroplasty include femoral shaft

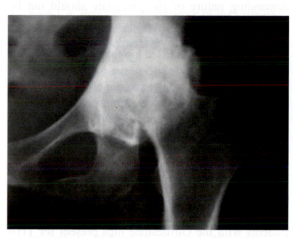

Figure 9: Old ankylosed hip (post-tuberculosis)

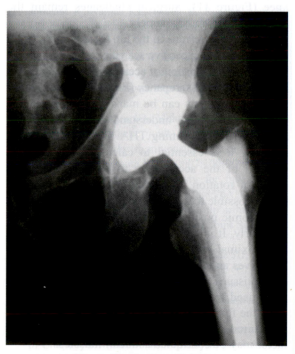

Figure 10: Postoperative THA

18. Kim YY, Ko Cu, Ahn JY, Yoon YS, Kwak BM. Charnley low friction arthroplasty in tuberculosis of the hip—an 8 to 13 year follow-up. J Bone Joint Surg Br 1988;70:756-60.

19. Laforgia R, Murphy JCM, Red-fern TR. Low friction arthroplasty for old quiescent infection of the hip. J Bone Joint Surg (Br) 1988;70B:373-6.

20. Liscomb PR, McCaslin FE Jr. Arthrodesis of the hip review of 371 cases. J Bone Joint Surg (Am) 1961 43A:923-79.

21. Mariconda M, Cozzolino A, Attingenti P, Cozzolino F, Milano C. Osteoarticular tuberculosis in a developed country. J Infect 2007;54:375-80.

22. Masri BA, Duncan CP, Jewesson P, Ngui-Yen J, Smith J. Streptomycin-loaded bone cement in the treatment of tuberculosis osteomyelitis—an adjunct to conventional therapy. Can J Surg 1995;38:64-8.

23. McCullough CJ. Tuberculosis as a late complication of total hip replacement. Acta Orthop Scan 1977;48: 508-10.

24. Stinchfield FE, Cavallaro WU. Arthrodesis of the hip joint: a follow-up study. J Bone Joint Surg (Am) 1950;32:48-57.

25. Strathy Gregg M, Fitzgerald Robert H Jr. Total hip arthroplasty in the ankylosed hip. J Bone Joint Surg 1988;70A:963-6.

26. Tuli SM (Ed). Tuberculosis of the Skeletal system (Bones, Joints, Spine and Bursal Sheaths), 2nd edn. New Delhi, India: Jaypee Brothers Medical Publishers 1997.

27. Tuli SM, Mukherjee SK. Excision arthroplasty for tuberculous and pyogenic arthritis of the hip. J Bone Joint Surg (Br) 1981;63B:29-32.

28. Yoon TR, Rowe SM, Anwar IB, Chung JY. Active tuberculosis of the hip treated with early total hip replacement—a report of 3 cases. Acta Orthop Scand 2001;72:419-21.

29. Yoon TR, Rowe SM, Santosa SB, Jung ST, Seon JK. Immediate cement less total hip arthroplasty for the treatment of active tuberculosis. J Arthroplasty 2005;20:923-26.

10 | Total Hip Replacement in Ankylosing Spondylitis

JA Pachore, HR Jhunjhunwala, Vikram I Shah, Sachin G Gujarathi

Ankylosing spondylitis is a member of a group of rheumatic diseases that affect the mobility of the spine, collectively known as spondyloarthropathies. The disease is characterized by axial skeletal involvement (sacroilitis, spines, ribs and sternum) and also involvement of peripheral joints (hip, shoulder, hands and feet). Peripheral major joint arthritis can occur soon after clinical presentation of axial skeletal disease.[1] Hip causes symptoms in 25-50% of patients, out of which 50-90% have bilateral involvement.[2,3]

The symptoms of this disease start in late adolescent and early childhood which is productive part of the life. The diagnosis is unacceptably delayed between onset and the diagnosis. The reported average interval may be between 8 and 11 years.[4] Patients presenting with clinical picture of ankylosing spondylitis before the age of 15 years are usually labeled as juvenile ankylosing spondylitis. Fifteen percent of this group of patients will need total hip replacement. On the other hand, the patients who present after 20 years of age, only 1% of them may have to undergo total hip replacement.

The treatment with early diagnosis has changed the management course for the betterment of the patient. Nonsteroidal anti-inflammatory drug is the main stay which controls the symptoms and may have protective effect on structural damage when used on regular basis.[5] Though NSAIDs and DMARDs have prominent effect on peripheral joint involvement, they have limited effect on the spine. TNF α and antigens of some strains of *Klebseilla* have been associated with ankylosing spondylitis.[6] Anti-tumor necrosis factor (Anti-TNF α) have prompt and robust effect on almost all aspects of the active disease. Patients have excellent pain relief, functional outcome, spinal mobility, peripheral arthritis and enthisitis, improved bone density and reduction of acute inflammation as seen on MRI images with anti-TNF α therapy.[7] No definite cure is available yet.

HISTORY

This disease was recognized by Galon as early as 17th century AD which was different than rheumatoid arthritis.[8] The skeletal evidence of bamboo spine in archeological skeleton remains of 5000 years Egyptian mummies have been documented. The neurophysiologist Vladimir Bekhterev of Russia in 1893, Adolf Strumpell of Germany in 1897 and Pierre Marie of France in 1898 were the first to give adequate description of the disease which allowed the accurate diagnosis.[9-11] Hence, this disease is named as Bekhterev disease or Marie-Strumpell disease.

Laboratory Studies

The diagnosis of ankylosing spondylitis is mostly clinico-radiological, however, laboratory findings have supportive role in establishing the same.
1. Elevated ESR and CRP are found in 75% of the patients and these are used as therapeutic as well as disease activity markers.[12]
2. Alkaline phosphatase and creatine kinase (CK) may be elevated but values are not useful as diagnostic or disease activity marker.

3. This spondyloarthropathy is associated with presence of a genetic marker called as HLA-B27. HLA-B27 is present in most of these patients; also the direct relationship between ankylosing spondylitis and HLA-B27 has been determined. However, its presence is not necessary to establish the diagnosis.[13] There are eleven subtypes of HLA-B27. Out of these four are strongly associated with ankylosing spondylitis viz B2702, B2704, B2705 and B2706. In South India HLA-B27 is positive in 83% of ankylosing spondylitis patients while it is positive in 94% of ankylosing patients in North India.[14,15]

4. Mean platelet volume (MPV) is a new marker under investigation for inflammatory pathologies. It is found to be significantly low in patients with ankylosing spondylitis and rheumatoid arthritis relative to control group. Also this value increases significantly after the therapy.[16]

Radiology

Early involvement of sacroiliac joint is hallmark of the disease. The earliest sign is fuzziness of sacroiliac joint (indistinctness). The joint space widens initially, then slowly narrows and progressively fusion takes place. Subchondral bone lesions are seen more on iliac side, followed by sclerosis and bony proliferation. The involvement is bilateral and symmetrical and as fusion takes place the sclerosis resolves. The bilateral sacroilitis may be found in other conditions like psoriasis, Reiter's disease, enteropathic arthropathy, hyperparathyroidism and osteitis condensans ilii.

The spinal involvement in early stage shows small erosion at the corner of vertebral bodies called as shiny corner sign or 'Romanus lesion'. The squaring of the vertebrae is characteristic feature of this disease. This is best seen in lumbar spine. The periosteal new bone formation occurs at the corner of the vertebrae followed by syndesmophyte formation. This is nothing but ossification of outer fibers of annulus fibrosus. The syndesmophyte fuses anteriorly with adjacent paravertebral tissues. Posterior interspinous ligament ossification produces a dense sclerotic line in midline. The apophyseal and the costovertebral joints initially show erosion followed by fusion. Complete fusion of vertebrae and all around tissue looks like bamboo spine. Calcification of disks at one or multiple level may be seen. Occasionally pseudoarthrosis at discovertebral area with destruction and adjacent sclerosis is seen and this lesion is called as 'Andersson lesion'. These are often misdiagnosed as infective lesions. The pseudoarthrosis is due to either an old missed fracture or an old unfused segment. And hence these patients need surgical stabilization.

Enthesopathy is seen as ill defined erosions with adjacent sclerosis at the site of ligamentous and tendinous attachments. These are usually bilateral and commonly seen at the ischial tuberosity, iliac crest and femoral trochanter.

Hip involvement as synovitis shows marked vascularity, hyperplasia of linning layer, lymphoid infiltration and pannus formation. Subchondral granulation tissue causes central cartilaginous erosion.[17] Osteoporosis occurs on both sides of the joint with synovitis. The cortical margins become indistinct and gradually the joint space narrows. The surface erosion starts leading to damage of the articular cartilage. There is always concentric joint space reduction which is characteristic feature of this disease, rheumatoid arthritis and few other inflammatory pathologies. Bony ankylosis takes place in around 24% of the patients. Very small percentage (7%) may go for protrusion. And the remaining proportion of patients present as chondrolytic variety.

Radiological Classification of Hip Pathology

The radiological classification (Figures 1A to C) has been described by Dr K T Dholakia et al. Three types have been described:[18]

1. Chondrolytic – concentric reduction of the joint space with involvement of articular cartilage. This corresponds to 69% of the patients.
2. Ankylosis – bony trabeculae crossing across the joint line, which correspond to 24%.
3. Protrusio – which is less common. Occurs in 7% of the patients.

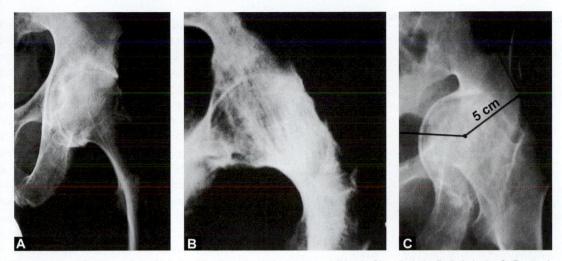

Figures 1A to C: The radiological classification of ankylosing spondylitis: A. Chondrolytic; B. Ankylosis; C. Protrusio

Medical Comorbidities in Ankylosing Spondylitis

Extra-articular manifestations are common in ankylosing spondylitis. Most common being acute anterior uveitis which occurs in 25 to 30% of patients.[19] Up to 60% of patients have inflammatory bowel disease which is usually asymptomatic. Frank inflammatory bowel disease occurs in 5 to 10% patients. Ten percent of patients may also have psoriatic features. Few percentage of patients have aortic insufficiency, worsening to congestive cardiac failure. Third degree heart block may occur in patients of ankylosing spondylitis.[17] These particular comorbities are important to recognize for smooth and safe perioperative management.

Anesthesia Consideration

Due to stiff or bamboo spine it is difficult to have access for spinal or combined spinal and epidural anesthesia. Lateral paraspinal approach for spinal anesthesia is preferred by many anesthetists but can be failure in a severely ankylosed spine. Routine intubation may not be possible in stiff or ankylosed cervical spine with temporomandibular joint involvement. Some of the patients need fiberoptic intubation for general anesthesia. Patients do need pulmonary function tests and blood gases preoperatively. The cardiopulmonary function is compromised in these patients, hence, preoperative anesthetist check up and counseling is helpful.

Indications of Total Hip Arthroplasty

Total hip arthroplasty is well established procedure with predictable results in ankylosing spondylitis. The main indication remains:

1. Painful hip interfering with daily living activities.
2. Deformity interfering with daily living activities.
3. Stiff hip or ankylosed hip in nonfunctional position (Figures 2A and B).
4. Social reasons.

When hip and spine both get involved, the hip pathology should be tackled first. Most of the spinal deformities get fairly corrected after hip replacement and do not require any corrective spinal osteotomy. Few patients may need spinal osteotomy after total hip arthroplasty and it is easier to determine the desired correction of the spine. Almost all authors agree that hip deformity should be corrected before spinal osteotomy.[20]

SURGICAL TECHNIQUE

Position of patient in ankylosing spondylitis is crucial due to deformed spine and fixed pelvic deformity;

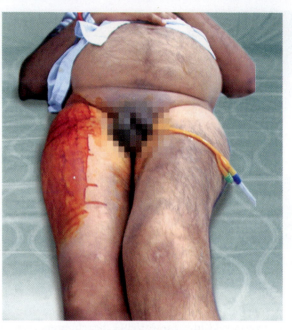

Figure 2A: Clinical picture: ankylosis in nonfunctional position

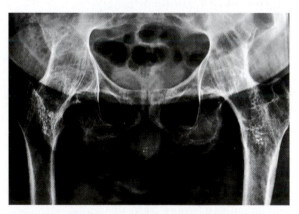

Figure 2B: Radiograph of the patient in figure 2A: Bilateral ankylosis of hip

patients with fixed external rotation and abduction deformities anterolateral or transtrochanteric approach can be a better choice. In patients with bony ankylosis surgeon should be prepared for trochanteric osteotomy or dual approach if neck is not visualized during the exposure. Once the neck is visualized, the osteotomy is done approximately 2 cm above the lesser trochanter (Caution—avoid cutting into greater trochanter or dividing posterior acetabular wall). Efforts should be made to leave a spike of bone at the superolateral acetabular margin. This allows containment of the cup and avoids the vertical position of it. Do not do higher osteotomy which may lead to an uncontained cup. The dual approach includes initial posterior approach with release of external rotators. If neck is not visible, through the same incision the anterior exposure is done between gluteus medius and vastus lateralis. Anterior capsule is exposed and incised along the neck, followed by two spikes to be introduced around the neck and the neck osteotomy is to be done. Rest of the procedure is done through posterior approach. After surgery both the approaches are closed in routine fashion. Chondrolytic variety of ankylosing spondylitis has a lot of inflammatory synovitis which leads to pain and spasm. All patients of this variety are practically stiff and painful preoperatively, however, after anesthesia pain and spasm gets relieved leading to smooth dislocation of femoral head intraoperatively.

Protrusio variety of ankylosing spondylitis should be treated like rheumatoid protrusio. The careful posterior exposure, capsular release and gentle gradual rotation for dislocation must be done. In case of difficult dislocation, some degree of posteroinferior lip of acetabulum(2-4 mm) can be taken off before the dislocation. If dislocation is not possible even with this, one should do neck osteotomy *in situ*. And the head can be taken out in piecemeal manner.

Acetabulum preparation is done with gentle reaming in all three varieties of ankylosing spondylitis. Special care has to be taken in ankylosed variety. After the neck osteotomy start reaming with small reamer at 90 degrees to transverse plane and this has to be gentle as the bone is extremely osteoporotic (Figure 3). Power reamers should be used with caution. The medial wall is seen by

hence, it is mandatory for a surgeon to position their patients personally. Surgeon must assess the range of motion after anesthesia (except in ankylosed hip), this will guide him for the approach and anticipation of dislocation difficulties.

The surgical approach depends on surgeons training, experience and the deformities. The

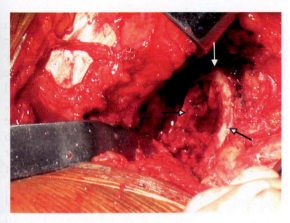

Figure 3: Acetabular view after femoral neck osteotomy in ankylosed hip (before reaming)

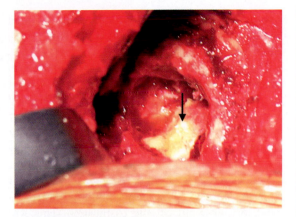

Figure 4: Acetabular view after reaming over neck osteotomy: The 'Fat Pad Sign'

presence of pulvinar pad of fat. Once the fat is seen, it indicates the most medial wall of the acetabulum. This pad of fat is the constant finding in spontaneous ankylosed hip. This finding we would like to document as 'Fat pad sign' (Figure 4). Many authors have vaguely described the pulvinar pad of fat in this pathology. However, we are describing this pad of fat in spontaneous bony ankylosis in eighty cases of ankylosing spondylitis. In all the cases the fat pad sign was positive; however, the amount of fat seen was variable. As this pad of fat does not get burnt out in this pathology. The rest of the reaming has to be done in routine fashion. One may rely on transverse acetabular ligament as an inferior landmark for anteversion of the cup which has been described by Beverland.[21] Preference of the cup is uncemented, however it can be left to the philosophy of the surgeon.

The protrusio variety need gentle mouth reaming with gradually progressive reamers, similar to the technique used in rheumatoid protrusio. Do not ream the medial wall which is usually thin and sclerotic. The depth of the medial wall can be assessed by drill followed by depth gauge measurement. The dome of acetabulum should be reamed cautiously with small reamer just to take out fibrous tissue and remaining cartilage so as to expose some degree of subchondral bone. In these cases we do not expect good subchondral bleeding bone. With flexible 3.2 mm drill point multiple drill holes can be made

in the area of dome to expose subchondral bone. Protrusio need medial grafting depending on the grade. The graft used in patients own femoral head and the size of the graft are 2-3 mm thick and about one cm long like matchsticks. The graft should be impacted with impacter. The uncemented cup is the choice of implant in these cases. Most protrusio have anterior and posteroinferior osteophytes which need to be removed or else it may lead to impingement and/or dislocation postoperatively. These osteophytes should be removed with a trial liner *in situ* or after final implantation of acetabular cup. Majority of uncemented cups in protrusio need supplementary screws. The principle of protrusio is to restore normal center of rotation, strengthening of medial wall and lateralization of the cup.[22]

Femoral canals in ankylosing spondylitis are Dorr type "C" canal as a common finding. Regarding preparation of femoral canal the procedure is similar to any other pathology with a note of the canal being wider in ankylosing spondylitis. The choice of femoral stem is the surgeon's preference and his philosophy. The cemented stem in these group of patients have done extremely well. However, the wider canal necessitates two packets of cement, in spite of this one may not achieve without cementing (grade A). The reason for this is inadequate cancellous bone. Our experience of cemented stem has been low aseptic loosening in spite of 1st and 2nd generation cementing technique. The uncemented stems also have done well. However, one must keep in mind regarding broader femoral canal (Dorr type "C") , which may need fully coated stem.

The extent of soft tissue release required in ankylosing spondylitis is much more than any other hip pathology as these patients do not have good elasticity of the tissues. In our experience, majority of patients need iliopsoas release and adductor tenotomy. Gluteus maximus release is done routinely as a part of exposure which helps to put the anterior swan neck retractor or cobra retractor for acetabular exposure. Wound wash with pulsatile lavage is mandatory to avoid ectopic ossification. This was emphasized by Prof. George Bently, Prof. Robert Owen and Duthie.[23] Routine closure of posterior capsule is to be done by Ranawat's pull through suture technique which will avoid postoperative dislocation. Our experience shows rate of dislocation is low as compared to total hip arthroplasty done for other pathologies. An explanation which we can suggest is that, these patients do not have excellent hip mobility due to inherent problems of soft tissue.

Postoperatively these patients are put on capsule indomethacin 25 mg three times a day for six weeks to avoid ectopic ossification. There is good evidence to support indomethacin in various studies. The indomethacin must be started next day morning as osteoblastic reaction starts within 24 hours. The role of radiation has excellent supportive literature to avoid ectopic ossification. The radiation should be used within 24 hours of surgery. Type of radiation should be linear accelerator which avoids implant irradiation (Figure 5). The radiation is given only to the capsule by this technique. There are no detrimental adverse effects noted on bony in-growth or longitivity of the implant. The single dose of radiation should be 700 rads (350 rads from the anteroposterior and 350 rads from posteroanterior side) within 24 to 48 hours postoperative (Figures 6 and 7). We have an experience of this technique with 15 cases having satisfactory results (Figures 8 and 9). Our indication remains patients with ankylosed hip who are not in reproductive age group.

POSTOPERATIVE PROTOCOL

The cemented hips can start walking full weight bearing with walker after drain removal in either

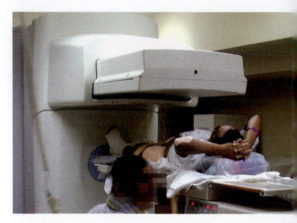

Figure 5: Linear accelerator for radiation prophylaxis of ectopic ossification

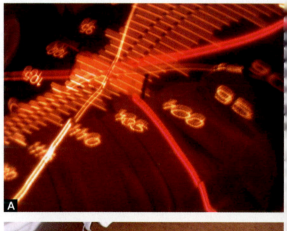

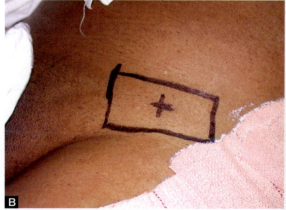

Figures 6A and B: Pre-radiation planning: A. Laser localization of capsular area to be irradiated; B. Marking for site of irradiation

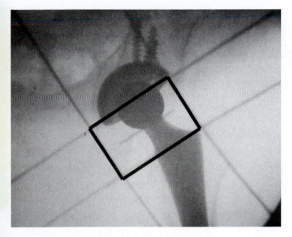

Figure 7: Grid for specific localized irradiation of capsular region: Image during radiotherapy

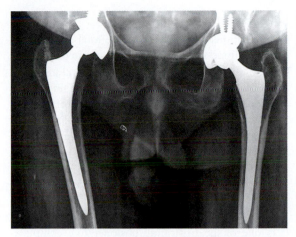

Figure 8: Three years follow-up with postoperative radiation prophylaxis showing no ectopic ossification

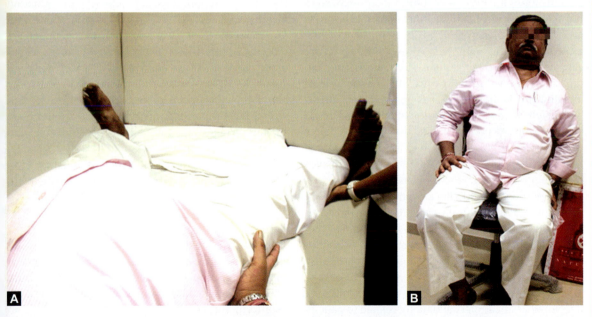

Figures 9A and B: Postoperative range of motion after total hip arthroplasty in the patient with bilateral ankylosis of hip

24 or 48 hours. Patients are discharged between 5th and 7th day. The uncemented hip has to walk partial weight bearing with walker for six weeks, followed by full weight bearing for another six weeks. At the end of three months they can have one stick on opposite side till they are comfortable or there is marked reduction in abductor limp. The ankylosed hip needs support while walking for a period of six months to one year postoperatively as abductors have to regain their strength. There is well documented evidence which states that, if nerve endplate is intact, the abductors will improve in course of time.

Complications

Complications concerned with the total hip replacement like infection, dislocation, deep vein thrombosis (DVT), thromboembolic phenomenon and mortality are similar to any other primary pathology. The rate of dislocation in ankylosing spondylitis is low; however, they have an unusual anterior dislocation even with posterior approach. Ectopic ossification being a unique complication related to ankylosing spondylitis is discussed.

Ectopic Ossification

It is one of the frustrating postoperative complications. The incidence of ectopic ossification varies in various studies with highest reported incidence being 61.7% by Bisla and Ranawat.[3] Various classifications are used to document their ossification but the most acceptable classification is Brooker et al. The cause of heterotopic ossification is not clearly understood. Many authors have suggested the cause can be hemorrhage, trauma, local inflammation, migration of bone marrow cells, and change in local metabolism. Mollon (1979) has reported that patients with high preoperative Serum alkaline phosphate are three times more likely to develop heterotopic ossification.[24] This complication is more common in males than females and this male predominance may suggest genetic predisposition. Patients with ossification on one side have overall 58% chance of developing ossification on opposite side. Ninety-six percent of the ossification is seen at 6 weeks as soft puffy callus. The maturation takes around 6 months, however, no additional ossification takes place after initial 6 weeks.[25]

Uncertainty that surrounds the issue of causation in ectopic ossification is undoubtly related to paucity of treatment modalities that exist for this problem today. Biphosphonates have been tried with limited success. Bentley and Duthie (1973) suggested that local irrigation of the wound with saline is useful in removing bone fragments which may stimulate osteogenesis around the prosthesis.[23] During 1970s numerous Scandinavian authors have investigated prostaglandin synthesis inhibitor like indomethacin. This is the drug of choice today and it should be started within 24 hours of the surgery and should be continued with the dose of 25 mg three times a day for 6 weeks. This drug does not hamper the osteointegration of uncemented implants. In 1974, Dahl reported considerable reduction of ectopic ossification with comparative study in a placebo group.[26] Ritter in 1985 reported overall difference in ectopic ossification between pre-indomethacin patients 26% and post-indomethacin patients 10% which was statistically significant.[27] As mentioned earlier linear accelerator with a dose of 700 rads within 24 to 48 hours of surgery has been one of the modalities of preventing ectopic ossification. The linear accelerator gives radiation only to the capsular area without radiating the implant and bone interface. Sell et al. reported better efficacy of radiation therapy over NSAIDs for hetrotopic ossification prophylaxis.[28] Ectopic ossification may hamper the mobility of hip. The clinical data suggest that mild to moderate ossification like Brooker I and II may not significantly reduce the movements of the hip. The re-ankylosis has been reported in the literature but with a small percentage. There has been no literature support suggesting the ectopic ossification and component loosening association. May and Yeoman, in 1986 have reported small series of 36 paients (54 hip replacements) having 18% ectopic ossification, out of which 2% have significant ossification.[29]

Results

The results of total hip replacement in ankylosing spondylitis are promising. The newer modern cemented arthroplasty will still improve the result. The uncemented total hip replacement has not reached long-term follow-up; hence, it will be difficult to predict the results. The new bearing surfaces will be the future direction as these patients are young and with high demands. The reported wear rate with conventional poly is high. Hence, the new bearing surfaces like highly crossed linked polyethylene, ceramic on ceramic and metal on metal need test of time for long-term results.

The long-term follow-up of cemented arthroplasty by DH Sochart and ML Porter (Wrightinton) suggests, the reported survival rate at 22.7 year is 88% for femoral component and 74% for acetabular component. The average wear rate has been reported 0.12 mm/year.[2]

Atul Joshi et al. reported a large series of cemented arthroplasty in ankylosing spondylitis. The survival rate of femoral components is 93% at 10 years, 88.2% at 15 years and 85.3% at 27 years. For acetabular components reported survival rate in this series is 96.1% at 10 years, 92.5% at 15 years, and 74.2% at 27 years.[30] Both these reports from Writington group have been encouraging. It seems femoral cemented components have done much better than the acetabular components.

Sweeney et al. reported outcome of 340 patients undergoing total hip replacement in ankylosing spondylitis. The survival rate reported as 90% at 10 years, 78% at 15 years and 64% at 20 years.[31]

The comparative survival of cemented and uncemented had been reported by Tang et al. and the survival reported for cemented hip arthroplasty is 98.5% at 5 years, 96.8% at 10 years and 63.3% at 15 years. The uncemented overall results have follow-up of 11 years with 63.3% survival.[32] Suryabhan et al. reported the conversion of ankylosed hip to total hip arthroplasty in ankylosing spondylitis by using uncemented components. The overall revision rate was 14% for aseptic loosening at 8.5 years. Their conclusion suggested that patients with ankylosed hip preoperatively had no pain and 38% patients had some pain after surgery but their satisfaction level was high. Hence, they recommended preoperative counseling regarding postoperative pain is mandatory in conversion THR for ankylosed hips.[33]

Many reports suggest anterior dislocation in ankylosing spondylitis in spite of using post approach. The explanation suggested by most authors is excessive anteversion mainly acetabular and vertical placement of the Cup. Suryabhan et al. had an observation of excessive anteversion of the femoral neck anatomy. Also they observed pelvic hyperextension and high inclination angle of acetabular components with severe involvement of the hip in ankylosing spondylitis. They also reported that anterior dislocation was common.[32,33]

Our Experience of Total Hip Replacement in Ankylosing Spondylitis

Three hundred eighty eight hips were operated at Bombay Hospital in the unit of Prof. KT Dholakia in patients with ankylosing spondylitis, out of which 219 were cemented hips, 60 hybrid and 109 were uncemented. In our observation, female:male ratio with ankylosing spondylitis requiring hip arthroplasty is 1:10. Seventy one percent of hips were done for bilateral involvement. The average age of these patients undergoing hip arthroplasty is 34 years. Twelve percent of all the hip arthroplasties were done for ankylosing spondylitis. The 74 cemented hips were followed up on long-term basis for 12-22 years with average follow-up being 15.2 years (Figure 10). Amongst the complications the rate of infection was 1%, dislocation 0.5%, trochanteric nonunion 1.1% and ectopic ossification 29% (mainly grade I and II). The aseptic loosening on femoral side was 6.7% in spite of generation 1 and 2 cementing technique. Aseptic loosening on acetabular side was 40.5%. The acetabular loosening rate was high due to high wear rate (Figure 11). Our study confirms the average wear

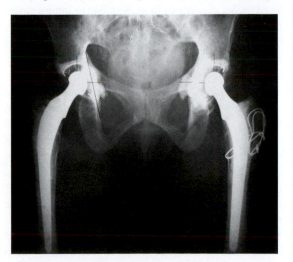

Figure 10: Twenty years follow-up in a patient with ankylosing spondylitis

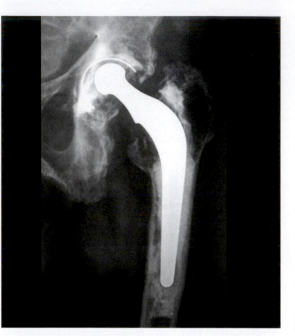

Figure 11: Osteolysis and wear in 22 years follow-up in ankylosing spondylitis

rate was 0.24 mm/year which was high as compared to other pathologies. Linear wear in the stable cup was 2.88 mm and loose cup it was 4.01 mm. This suggested the cups which have a high wear rate will have higher chances of loosening due to impingement phenomenon. This was well reported by Wroblewski.[34] Initially 1988 onwards till 1997 isoelastic uncemented hips were used which had high rate of stem loosening. In general we had 40% stem loosening at seventh year. This discouraged us to use this implant. From 1998 onwards we had used uncemented bicontact implant till today. In our observation of 43 hips with bicontact stem, none of the stem had aseptic loosening and not a single stem has been revised. On the acetabular side we have started noticing polywear and some degree of osteolysis. The wear reported is comparatively high in uncemented hips. There is a prospective randomized study done by Mc Combe P and William SA stating uncemented hips have 0.15 mm/year in contrast to cemented hips 0.7mm/year with $p < 0.0001$.[35] The long-term data for uncemented hips in ankylosing yet has not reached more than 15 years.

As we follow these patients on long-term then only we will have sufficient evidence to recommend cemented hips or uncemented hips. The new bearing surface in ankylosing spondylitis also does not have sufficient data to recommend what type of hip will last for life time! Past ten years more uncemented hips were done.

At Shalby hospital total fifty-two total hip arthroplasties were done in last three years for ankylosing spondylitis, among these fourteen patients were operated bilaterally. Uncemented technology was implemented in all these arthroplasties in last three years. Twenty patients required fiberoptic intubation which is fairly high number. The explanation which we can offer is this is a tertiary center and many patients are referred due to unavailability of fiberoptic facilities. There was no infection, dislocation or any perioperative morbidity or mortality in these patients.

AUTHORS' RECOMMENDATION

Work in close association with rheumatologist as to control the disease activity. Consider surgery only with fairly disabling patients. Ankylosed hips preoperative counseling will be needed to explain some degree of pain after the surgery but they will have benefit of mobility and function. These patients will also need a stick for a long time. Preoperative medical fitness in relation to cardiopulmonary function is required. The anesthetist should evaluate preoperatively to plan the type of anesthesia and the difficulties which he may encounter. Fiberoptic intubation has become a boon for this difficult cervical spine deformities. The position of the patient should be given under the observation of the surgeon. Surgical approach depends on deformity and surgeon's experience. Do not hesitate to do trochanteric osteotomy in a difficult ankylosed and protrusio hips. Under anesthesia most of the hips will have good movement and it is possible to dislocate the femoral head except ankylosed hips. In ankylosed hips neck osteotomy with caution and look for pad fat sign for medial wall of acetabulum while reaming. Uncemented hips are preferred. Intraoperative pulsatile lavage and postoperative indomethacin to avoid ectopic ossification.

REFERENCES

1. Forestier J, Lagier R. Ankylosing hyperostosis of spine. Clin Orthop Rel Research 1971;74:65-83.

2. Sochart DH, Porter ML. Long term results of total hip replacement in young patients who had ankylosing spondylitis. Eighteen to thirty year results with survivorship analysis. J Bone Joint Surg [Am] 1997;79(8):1181-9.

3. Bisla RS, Ranawat CS, Inglis AE. Total hip replacement in patients with ankylosing spondylitis with involvement of hip. J Bone Joint Surg [Am] 1976;58:233-8.

4. Feldtkeller E, Khan MA, Vander Heijde D, Vander Linden S, Braun J. Age at disease onset and diagnosis delay in HLA-B 27 negative v/s positive patients with ankylosing spondylitis. Rheumatol. Int. 2003;23:61-6.

5. Wander A, Vander Heijde D, Landewe R, et al. Nonsteroidal anti-inflammatory drug reduces radiographic presentation in patients with ankylosing spondylitis: a randomized clinical trial. Arthritis Rheum 2005;52:1756-65.

6. Rabindra Nath Sarkar, Kuntal Bhattacharyya, Sibaji Phaujdar, Dibendu De. Assessment of efficacy of pulse ibandronate therapy in nonsteroidal anti-inflammatory drug refractory ankylosing spondylitis. An Open Perspective Study. Indian J of Rheumatol 2011;6(2):55-60.

7. Sieper J, Rudwaleit M. Early referral recommendation for ankylosing spondylitis including preradiographic and radiographic normal in primary care. Ann Rheum Dis 2005;64:659-63.

8. Dieppe P, Dia Galon. Describe rheumatoid arthritis? Annals of Rheum Dis 1988;47(1):84-7.

9. Bechterew V, Steifigkeit der Wirbelsaale, Verkrummung als Besonaere Erkran Kungsform. Neurocentral b 1893;426-34.

10. Stumpell A. "Bemerkung uber disc chronicle. Ankylosirende Entzundung der Wribelsaule und der Huftgelenke". Dtsch 2 Nervenheilkd 1897;11:338-42.

11. Marie P. Shrla spondylose rhizomelique. Rev Med 1898;18:285-315.

12. RU of J , Stucki G. Validity aspect of ESR and C reactive protein in ankylosing spondylitis: a literature review J of Rheumatol Apr 1999;26(4):966-70.

13. Alvarez I, Lopez De Castro. HLA-B27 and immunogenetics of spondyloarthropathies. Curr Opin Rheumatol Jul 2000;12(4):248-53.

14. Radha Madhavan, Chandrashekharan AN, Paethiban M, et al. HLA profile of seronegative spondyloarthropathies in a referral hospital in South India. J Ind Rheum Assoc 1996;4:91-5.

15. Sanjeev Prakash, Mehta NK, Malaviya AN et al. Ankylosing spondylitis in North India – A clinical and immunogenetic study. Ann Rheum Dis 1984;43: 381-5.

16. Kisacik B, Tufan D, Kalyonca V, et al. Mean platelet volume as inflammatory marker in ankylosing spondylitis and rheumatoid arthritis. Joint Bone Spine 2008;75(3):291-4.

17. Joel D Taurog. The spondyloarthritides. 318 in Harrison's Principles of Internal Medicine. 17th Edition, edited by Fauci, Braunwald, Kasper, Hauser, Longo, Jameson, Loscazo. 2008;2:2109-13.

18. Total Hip Replacement in Ankylosing Spondylitis-Text Book - Joint Replacement. 'State of Art', 1990 - By Richard Coombs

19. Lt. Col. Achutan K, Porkodi R, Ramakrishnan S, et al. Pattern of rheumatic diseases in South India – Ankylosing spondylitis a clinical and radiological study. J Assoc Phy Ind 1990;38:10,774-7.

20. Camargo FP, Cordeiro EN, Napoli MM. Corrective osteotomy of the spine in Ankylosing spondylitis patients. Experience in 66 cases. Clin. Orthop 1986; 208:157.

21. Beverland D. The transverse acetabular ligament: optimizing version. Orthopaedics 2010;33(9): 631.

22. Ranawat CS, Zahn MG. Role of bone grafting in correction of protrusio acetabuli by total hip arthroplasty. J of Arthroplasty 1986;1(2):131-7.

23. Bentley G, Duthie RB. A comparative review of the Mckee Farrar and Charnley total hip prosthesis. Clin Orthop 1973;95:127-42.

24. Mollon RAB. Serum alkaline phosphatase in heterotopic para-articular ossification after total hip replacement. J Bone Joint Surg 1979;61(B):432-4.

25. Ritter MA, Vaughan RB. Ectopic ossification after total hip arthroplasty. J Bone Joint Surg. [Am] 1977;59(A):345-51.

26. Dhal HK. Kliniske Observasjoner. P-37. In Blindern MSD (Ed): Symposium on arthrose. MSD, Norway 1974;99:37.

27. Ritter MA , Sieber JM. Prophylactic indomethacin for prevention of heterotropic bone formation following total hip arthroplasty. Clin Orthop 1985;196:217-25.

28. Sell S, Willims R, Jany R, EsenWein S, Gaissmier

TOTAL HIP REPLACEMENT IN ANKYLOSING SPONDYLITIS

C, Martini F, et al. The suppression of heterotopic ossification. Radiation versus NSAID therapy a prospective study. J of Arthroplasty 1998;13(8): 854-9.

29. May PC, Yeoman PM. Hip arthroplasty in ankylosing spondylitis. J Bone Joint Surg 68(B);669.

30. Joshi Atul B, Markovic Ljnbisa, Hardinge Kevin, Murphy John CM. Total hip arthroplasty in ankylosing spondylitis. An analysis of 181 hips. J of Arthroplasty 2002;17(4):427-33.

31. Sweeney, Gupta R, Taylor G, Calin A. Total hip arthroplasty in ankylosing spondylitis: outcome in 340 patients. J of Rheumatology 2001;28(8):1862-6.

32. Tang WM, Chiu KY. Primary total hip arthroplasty in patients with ankylosing spondylitis. J of Arthroplasty 2000;15(1):52-58.

33. Suryabhan, Krishna Kiran Echampati, Rajesh Malhotra. Primary cementless THA for bony ankylosis in patients with ankylosing spondylitis. J of Arthroplasty 2008;33(6):859-66.

34. Wroblewski BM, Siney PD, Fleming PA. Wear of the cup in the Charnley LFA in the young patients. J Bone Joint Surg 2004;86(4):498-503.

35. Mc Combe P, Williams SA. A comparison of polyethylene wear rates between cemented and cementless cups. A prospective, randomized trial. J Bone Joint Surg Br 2004;86:344-9.

11 | Total Hip Arthroplasty in Patients with Neuromuscular Abnormalities

Rajiv Thukral, SKS Marya

INTRODUCTION

Patients with neuromuscular conditions like cerebral palsy, myelomeningocele, spinal injury, cerebrovascular accident (CVA), poliomyelitis, Parkinson's disease, Down's syndrome, spinal injury, etc. may need hip replacement for either of two reasons, for the disease process itself (rendering the hip dysplastic and secondarily arthritic), or for primary degenerative processes in the hip (as would occur in the rest of the population). Altered muscle tone (spastic or paralytic), and poor muscle control and coordination (including tremors and other involuntary movements) affect the performance of these hips in both the short-term (increased risk of dislocation, recurrence of contractures), and the long-term (loosening)[1,2] and so there are few studies reporting hip replacement in these conditions in literature. In addition to these limitations, rehabilitation is also fraught with complication and difficulty.[3]

However, with the advent of large femoral heads, improved surgical technique and instrumentation (including the use of pre- and intraoperative navigation to correctly predict and treat deformities and dysplasia), hip replacement is now being increasingly performed in patients with complex neuromuscular conditions who would have been previously managed with salvage procedures like excision/interposition arthroplasty or arthrodesis.[4-6]

Usually hip replacement in these patients is undertaken in a tertiary care hospital that specializes in these surgeries or who have large volumes of hip replacements as these patients are more prone to early failure.[4-7]

Because of these and other limitations (inability to assess outcomes by the usual scoring systems), few studies exist, and according to a review by Queally and Abdulkarim,[8] only 13 studies were accessible using the online medical literature search comprising Medline, EMBASE and Cochrane databases for articles between 1970 and 2009 that specifically dealt with this group of patients with respect to function, complications, surgical technique and postoperative management.

It is easy to divide patients with neuromuscular conditions into two groups for the purpose of understanding their management, possible complications and limitations. These include those with increased muscle tone and spasticity (exemplified by cerebral palsy, Parkinson's disease and post-CVA), and those with decreased muscle tone (exemplified by poliomyelitis, myelomeningocele, spinal injury). Also, each specific condition may be studied separately so as to identify their specific indications, surgical technique, possible complications and limitations.

Conditions with Increased Muscle Tone

These include cerebral palsy, Parkinson's disease and some cases of CVA.

Cerebral Palsy

Hip pain commonly affects 25 to 75% of patients,[9] and occurs as a result of dysplasia, subluxation, dislocation and osteoarthritis. Muscle imbalance and bony deformities predispose the femoral head to subluxate/dislocate, and there is subsequent gradual deformity and degeneration.[10] Treatment options for a painful degenerative adult hip joint here include resection, arthrodesis and replacement arthroplasty. Resection arthroplasty, with or without interposition techniques, requires extensive release to be effective, and is therefore reserved for patients with limited functional needs (of improved hygiene and better positioning). Arthrodesis is again indicated only in the immobile patient, and becomes a non-viable option if there is a co-existent spinal and/or contralateral hip deformity.

Total hip arthroplasty (THA) offers the best chance of pain relief and mobility. However, concerns of abnormal muscle tone, spasticity, contractures and patient compliance exist and have to be balanced against the advantages of low demand (reduced physical activity) and therefore longevity of the prosthesis, and must be taken into consideration while planning such a procedure. It must also be understood that standardized hip scores (like the Harris Hip score) cannot be used to describe outcomes in these patients, and results are more logically assessed by pain relief and walking status achieved postoperatively.

THA in painful hips of patients with cerebral palsy was first reported by Buly et al., as late as in 1993,[11] though since then some researchers have reported successful outcomes in certain groups of patients.[8,12,13] Buly et al.[11] showed good results (in terms of pain relief, rates of revision and functional improvement) at ten years in seventeen of eighteen patients using the cemented THA (prosthetic survival rate of 95%), though, of them, two had recurrent dislocations and sixteen patients needed postoperative immobilization in a spica cast. They used customized femoral implants, with tenotomies of contracted muscles, and placed the acetabular components in anteversion. Weber and Cabanela[12] treated patients of hemiplegia, diplegia, quadriplegia, athetoid quadriplegia and athetoid diplegia with cemented/hybrid THA, with thirteen of fifteen patients demonstrating pain relief. Complications included one case each of trochanteric avulsion, heel ulcer (post-spica cast) and urinary retention. Three patients needed re-surgery, but only

one of these was for a failed primary hip, that too 13 years after the index procedure. Blake et al.[13] treated a 14-year old patient with a painful dislocated hip with a constrained hybrid THA, with pain-free movements persisting at 2½ years follow-up. Queally and Abdulkarim[8] performed cementless THA in their patients. They managed dysplastic acetabula with careful templating, preoperative planning and intraoperative bone grafting as indicated. They mobilized the patient on post-operative day one, as they used constrained liners in 4 of 6 patients (who showed soft-tissue imbalance) and 'stem-and-sleeve' femoral designs (for 4 patients with abnormal proximal femoral anatomy. Postoperative contractures were tackled with a combination of surgical and botulinum toxin release. At one year, their results matched those seen by others[10-12] even though they used cementless components.

All these studies clearly indicate that though there are intraoperative difficulties that need to be taken care of and postoperative complications that may arise, with modified surgical techniques and appropriate implant choice, good outcomes are achievable with THA.

Parkinson's Disease

Musculoskeletal effects of Parkinson's disease include tremors, rigidity, contractures, bradykinesia, dystonia, and postural instability, and all of these contribute to the morbidity in addition to the hip pathology, with theoretical increased risk of dislocation of the hip.[14] Modern medical treatment has been very successful in reducing the tremors, rigidity and akinesia seen in patients with Parkinson's disease, and this has substantially helped tackle the biggest postoperative challenges after THA in these patients. Indications have included fractures, arthritis and avascular necrosis. Impairment of balance and righting reflexes, and postural hypotension associated with medication may create difficulty in the postoperative period, and high complication rates (and unsatisfactory results) and increased mortality has been seen in many reports over time.[15-18] Further, even though the initial results were good in terms of functional recovery and ability to walk without aids in a large majority, most patients deteriorated over time due to the natural progression of the disease, thus producing poor end-results at longer follow-up.[14,18,19] High mortality rates of 20-47% have been reported at six months,[17,20] with complications in up to 26% of patients (incl. wound infection, dislocation, deep vein thrombosis, urinary tract infections, pneumonia and postoperative confusion) for patients with femoral neck fractures.[17,19] High rates of re-operation for different reasons[19,20] including deep wound infection, periprosthetic fracture, trochanteric nonunion, aseptic loosening, late instability, etc. have further deterred the arthroplasty surgeon from giving a good prognosis in these patients.[20]

Pain relief has, however, been seen unfailingly to be successful following THA for any cause (femoral neck fractures, osteoarthritis, failed endoprostheses, aseptic loosening) in patients with Parkinson's disease.[18-20]

Weber et al.[20] in their series of 28,000 THAs performed over 24 years (1970-1994) found that 98 (0.4%) were done for various causes in patients with Parkinson's disease. At a mean follow-up of 7.1 years, using both cemented and cementless components, though functional outcomes improved in the early follow-up period, 57% deteriorated with progression of the neurological condition, and 26% had some postoperative complication. Similarly, Meek et al.[3] reported the findings of the Scottish National Arthroplasty Registry. Out of 14,314 THAs done between 1996 and 2004, they found that Parkinson's affected 5-8% of patients. Although other authors have reported high dislocation rates, they found that dislocation rates were significantly lower in these patients vis-à-vis control groups,[3] and they contributed this due to appropriate medical management for the neurological symptoms. Abdul-karim et al.[8] share the same philosophy, and always place emphasis on the preoperative control of the neurological disorder, and postoperative medical management to avoid complications. Cabanela and Weber[12,19] have concluded that though the prevalence of complications (particularly dislocation and higher rates of infection) in patients with Parkinson's disease is relatively high, attention to technical detail (including judicious use of adductor and psoas tenotomy in the presence of severe contractures) is paramount. A higher mortality rate may be expected in the first six months after THA, and progression of Parkinson's is the rule, and therefore even though pain relief is good, functional outcomes deteriorate rapidly overtime.

CVA (Stroke)

Unfortunately there is very little evidence in literature that reports the outcomes of THA in patients suffering from a history of cerebrovascular accidents (CVA). Traditionally considered high risk for dislocation (due to contractures and muscle atrophy), the findings of the Scottish National Registry by Meek et al.[3] (suggesting an annual incidence of 2 to 6% of CVA in patients undergoing THA) state a rate of dislocation lower than the control group, attributed to possible reduced mobility in these patients. Heterotopic ossification (HO) has been seen to occur with increased incidence in patients recovering from stroke, and this has been substantiated by DiCaprio et al.[21] in their series of 31 THAs in 22 patients, who showed rates of 36% compared to 15% in controls. They now recommend routine radiation prophylaxis for HO prevention in patients with history of CVA undergoing THA. This pattern of increased HO is also seen in patients with spinal injury (with tetraplegia or paraplegia), as reported by Becker et al.[22] A small number of paraplegic patients with functional disability and pain (secondary osteoarthritis) have been treated by THA by Abdulkarim et al.[8] with good functional and pain relief measures. Risk of dislocation prompted the use of constrained implants.[8] Constrained liners have reported to provide stability in patients with neurologic diseases, though may aggravate loosening, as demonstrated in a comparative study by Hernigou et al.[23]

Conditions with Decreased Muscle Tone

These include poliomyelitis, myelomeningocele, Down's syndrome, tabes dorsalis and neuropathic joints.

Poliomyelitis

Although successful polio vaccination has almost eliminated acute poliomyelitis, many patients all over the world suffer sequelae of this viral infection, with residual lower limb paralysis, deformities and degenerative joint disease. Some of the common bone and soft tissue problems of these patients include dysplasia of the acetabula, subluxation, contractures, poor bone quality, femoral head abnormalities (coxa valga, excessive anteversion), pelvic obliquity, leg length discrepancy, contractures and limb atrophy. Pelvic obliquity, in addition to muscular imbalance and contractures contribute to subluxation and instability, and this obliquity may sometimes result from contralateral hip adduction/abduction contractures.[24]

The THA is rarely used to treat degenerative hip disease in patients with old residual poliomyelitis deformities. A few case reports exist in literature. Laguna and Barrientos[25] used cementless components with acetabular bulk allograft (with lowering of the hip center) to treat an osteoarthritic dysplastic hip in a 38-year-old female with flaccid paralysis secondary to poliomyelitis. Spinnickie and Goodman[26] used a constrained THA for treatment of nonunion of the femoral neck fracture in a 71-year-old man with residual polio deformity, and Cameron[27] also has reported a similar case with good function and pain scores at 3 years follow-up. Cabanela et al.[19] have 2 to 8 year results in 5 patients that appear no different from that in the general population.

Myelomeningocele

The problem with myelomeningocele is that paralysis of the hip muscles does not permit useful function even after hip replacement for painful dysplasia of the hip. Weber and Cabanela[19] found 3 patients with low-lumbar-level myelomeningocele who had THA because of hip pain. However, all the prostheses performed poorly due to persistent pain and instability at a follow-up of 5 to 10 years.[19] They concluded that THA should be reserved only for patients who have symptomatic arthritis without neuropathic arthropathy, and with adequate muscle control, while the rest should be managed by arthrodesis or excision.

Queally and Abdulkarim have recommended the use of constrained liners, though with the caveat of keeping the possibility of component dissociation in mind.[8]

Down's Syndrome

THA is sometimes indicated in these patients because of hip dysplasia with secondary osteoarthritis. A search of the Mayo Joint Registry confirmed 5 THAs for painful dysplastic hips in 3 patients of Down's syndrome. Cemented implants fared well at 5 to 15 years follow-up, while cementless implants had been revised due to loosening.[19] There were no episodes of dislocation or any other complication otherwise, and this would seem to suggest that when properly indicated, cemented total hip arthroplasty performs reasonably well in patients with Down's syndrome, as the muscular disorder is minimal.

Tabes Dorsalis and Charcot's Arthritis

The THA has been used very rarely in Charcot's arthropathy of the hip, though it is a contraindication. Sprenger and Foley[30] described a successful THA in one patient, and attributed this to absent ataxia in their patient. Robb et al.[29] on the other hand, described multiple recurrent dislocations after one such instance in a 58-year-old female with history of Tabes dorsalis, whose implants were finally removed after numerous unsuccessful attempts at open reduction and soft tissue reconstruction.

DISCUSSION

Total hip arthroplasty THA in patients with neuromuscular conditions presents special challenges. The anatomy is abnormal, with varying degrees of structural and functional complex compensatory mechanisms at play. Altered acetabular anatomy, orientation and function (dysplasia, excessive anteversion, subluxation, dislocation, microacetabuli), altered femoral anatomy, orientation and function (coxa valga, excessive anteversion, malrotation, flexion and adduction/abduction contractures), movement disorders (ataxia, tremors, abnormal movements, etc.) and pelvic and spinal deformities (pelvic obliquity, truncal imbalance, proximal and distal muscle weakness/paralysis or spasticity) all contribute in various degrees to the complexity of the situation. A proper understanding and assessment of this is essential prior to undertaking a hip replacement procedure in these conditions.

Next up, the proper indications must be understood and contraindications well-defined. Pain and disability must be severe enough to justify hip arthroplasty in these patients.

Before surgery, proper preoperative planning as to the surgical approach, need for alternate approaches (trochanteric osteotomies, combined releases, corrective osteotomies and tenotomies) must be anticipated. Appropriate implant systems with modular components must be available as anatomy is altered. Present day availability of large bearings, customized and modular pressfit cups and stems, and constrained acetabular liners have minimized the risk of dislocations and postoperative loosening. Forces that otherwise would have been contributing to dislocation have been transferred to the locking mechanism of the constrained liners and liner-shell and shell-bone interfaces,[13] producing success rates of up to 98% at 4.8 years follow-up in managing recurrent instability.[23,31] Similarly, use of stem-and-sleeve constructs can address complex femoral anatomy, in particular problems with anteversion, metaphyseal-diaphyseal mismatch, and reduced lateral and vertical offset; which cannot be accommodated by standard off-the-shelf monoblock or even modular implants.

Postoperative complications must be anticipated, prepared for and adequately treated. Appropriate tenotomies, releases, use of postoperative bracing and splinting, and appropriate prolonged antibiotics (as in Parkinson's disease) would be instituted. Patients with contractures or muscle weakness need corrective methods (surgically and pharmaceutically).

Another point that needs to be understood and accepted is that THA in these patients gives reliably good outcome in pain relief, function and walking ability, though this has the limitation of not being standardized to routine hip scoring systems. Radiographic assessment may be carried out routinely, though the main parameters for outcome need to be pain and walking ability.

As medical management of these neurological conditions improve, these patients will live longer and are more likely to need hip arthroplasty for symptomatic arthritis. Current evidence suggests that contemporary THA using modular implants, constrained components (when required), soft-tissue releases (when appropriate) and a multi-disciplinary approach to management should be considered in these severely disabled patients. In conclusion, THA can give good outcomes in the medium-term to these patients with neuromuscular disorders.

REFERENCES

1. Espehaug B, Havelin LI, Engesaeter LB, Langeland B, Vollset SE. Patietn related risk factors for early revision of total hip replacements: a population register-based case-control study of 674 revised hips, Acta Orthop Scand 1997;68:207-15.
2. Paterno SA, Lachiewicz PF, Kelley S. The influence of patient-related factors and the position of the acetabular component on the rate of dislocation after total hip replacement. J Bone Joint Surg [Am] 1997;79-A:1202-10.
3. Meek RM, Allan DB, McPhillips G, Kerr L, Howie CR. Epidemiology of dislocation after total hip arthroplasty. Clin Orthop 2006;447:9-18.
4. Castle ME, Schneider C. Proximal femoral resection-interposition arthroplasty. J Bone Joint Surg [Am] 1978;60-A:1051-4.
5. Root L, Goss JR, Mendes J. The treatment of the painful hip in cerebral palsy by total hip replacement or hip arthrodesis. . J Bone Joint Surg [Am] 1986;68-A:590-8.
6. Koffman M. Proximal femoral resection or total hip replacement in cerebral palsy: long-term follow-up results. Orthop Clin North Am 1981;12:91-100.
7. Woolson ST, Rahimtoola ZO. Risk factors for dislocation during the first 3 months after primary total hip replacement. J Arthroplasty 1999;14:662-8.
8. Queally JM, Abdulkarim A, Mulhall KJ. Total hip replacement in patients with neurological conditions. J Bone Joint Surg [Br] 2009;91-B:1267-73.
9. Bagg MR, Farber J, Miller F. Long-term follow-up of hip subluxation in cerebral palsy patients. J Paediatr Orthop 1993;13:32-6.
10. Moreau M, Drummond DS, Rogala E, Ashworth A, Porter T. Natural history of the dislocated hip in spastic cerebral palsy. Dev Med Child Neurol 1979; 21:749-53.

11. Buly RL, Huo M, Root L, Binzer T, Wilson PD Jr. Total hip arthroplasty in cerebral palsy. Long-term follow-up results. Clin Orthop1993;296:148-53.

12. Weber M, Cabanela ME. Total hip arthroplasty in patients with cerebral palsy. Orthopedics 1999;22:425-7.

13. Blake SM, Kitson J, Howell JR, Gie GA, Cox PJ. Constrained total hip arthroplasty in a paediatric patient with cerebral palsy and painful dislocation of the hip: a case report. J Bone Joint Surg [Br] 2006; 88-B:655-7.

14. Hoehn MM, Yahr MD. Parkinsonism: Onset, progression and mortality. Neurology 1967;17(5): 427-42.

15. Rothermel JE, Garcia A. Treatment of hip fractures in patients with Parkinson's disease on levodopa therapy. J Bone Joint Surg [Br] 1985;67-B(3):424-5.

16. Soto-Hall R. Treatment of transcervical fractures complicated by certain common neurological conditions. In Instructional Course Lectures, American Academy of Orthopaedic Surgeons. Vol 17, pp. 117-20. St. Louis, C.V. Mosby, 1960.

17. Staeheli JW, Frassica FJ, Sim FH. Prosthetic replacement of the femoral head for fracture of the femoral neck in patients who have Parkinson disease. J Bone Joint Surg [Am] 1988;70-A:565-8.

18. Turcotte R, Godin C, Duchesne R, Jodoin A. Hip fractures and Parkinson's disease. A clinical review of 94 fractures treated surgically. Clin Orthop 1990; 256:132-6.

19. Cabanela ME, Weber M. Total hip arthroplasty in patients with neuromuscular disease. J Bone Joint Surg [Am] 2000;82-A(3):426-32.

20. Weber M, Cabanela ME, Sim FH, Frassica FJ, Harmsen WS. Total hip replacement in patients with Parkinson's disease. Int Orthop 2002;26:66-8.

21. DiCaprio MR, Huo MH, Zatorski LE, Keggi K. Incidence of heterotopic ossification following total hip arthroplasty in patients with prior stroke. Orthopedics 2004;27:41-3.

22. Becker SW, Rohl K, Weidt F. Endoprosthesis in paraplegics with periarticular ossification of the hip. Spinal Cord 2003;41:29-33.

23. Hernigou P, Filippini P, Flouzat-Lachaniette CH, Batista SU, Poignard A. Constrained liner in neurologic or cognitively impaired patients undergoing primary THA. Clin Orthop Relat Res 2010; 20376709.

24. Delauney CP, Bonnomet F, Clavert P, Laffargue P, Migaud H. THA using metal-on-metal articulation in active patients younger than 50 years. Clin Orthop 2008;466:340-6.

25. Laguna R, Barrientos J. Total hip arthroplasty in paralytic dislocation form poliomyelitis. Orthopedics 2008;31:179.

26. Spinnickie a, Goodman SB. Dissociation of the femoral head and trunion after constrained conversion total hip arthroplasty for poliomyelitis. J Arthroplasty 2007;22:634-7.

27. Cameron HU. Total hip replacement in a limb severely affected by paralytic poliomyelitis. Can J Surg 1995;38:386.

28. Weber M, Cabanela. Total hip arthroplasty in patients with low-lumbar-level myelomeningocoele. Orthopedics 1998;21:709-12.

29. Robb JE, Rymaszewski LA, Reeves BF, Lacey CJ. Total hip replacement in a Charcot joint: brief report. J Bone Joint Surg [Br] 1988;70-B:489.

30. Sprenger TR, Foley CJ. Hip replacement in a Charcot joint: a case report and historical review. Clin Orthop 1982;165:191-4.

31. Su EP, Pellici PM. The role of constrained lines in total hip arthroplasty. Clin Orthop 2004;420:122-9.

12 | Total Hip Replacement in Dysplastic Hips

Vijay C Bose

Prosthetic replacement in a dysplastic hip is one of the most challenging forms of joint replacement surgeries. High complication and revision rates have been reported in the literature with these procedures. Though the abnormality is primarily in the shape of the acetabulum, the afflicted hips often have accompanying deformities of the proximal femur and the adjoining soft tissues. Both femoral and acetabular reconstructions are therefore complex in nature. This group of patients are usually young, very active and place high expectations from their reconstructed joints. A thorough understanding of the principles and the risks involved in reconstructing dysplastic joints becomes essential.

ANATOMY

In mild dysplasia, the subluxation is minimal and the pathology is limited to the acetabulum. In more severe afflictions associated with gross subluxation or frank dislocation of the femoral head, there is greater soft-tissue and bony anomalies. In such severe cases, the acetabular socket is hypoplastic as the head has never articulated with the acetabulum. The acetabulum has a high degree of anteversion, with anterior wall deficiency but a well-preserved posterior wall. The femur is also hypoplastic and its proximal end distorted. The femoral head is disproportionate with a large mediolateral (ML) diameter (Mushroom head), and the femoral neck is usually in valgus and anteverted. The greater trochanter is displaced posteriorly with accompanying weakness of the

abductors. The soft tissue structures are stretched and add to the laxity of the joint. The neurovascular structures may be displaced from their normal positions. This is important to keep in mind while performing releases during reconstruction of the joint.

Before proceeding with surgery, an assessment of the joint is necessary especially relating to the severity of the condition. A popular classification among the surgeons is Crowe's grading system.[1] This classification relies on the degree of femoral head displacement (Figures 1A to D and Table 1).

Table 1: Crowe's classification of dysplastic hips

Grade	Criteria
Grade 1	50%
Grade 2	50 – 75%
Grade 3	75 – 100%
Grade 4	Complete dislocation

Hartofilakadis[2] described another system of classifying dysplastic hips. They group the dysplastic hips into three basic types. The dysplastic group contains all the hips with the femoral heads contained within the acetabular sockets. The low displacement group consists of hips where the femoral head has migrated superiorly to articulate with a false acetabulum, but still maintains contact with the original acetabular socket. The third variety is the high dislocation type in which the femoral head in its entirety articulates with the ilium with no contact with the original acetabular

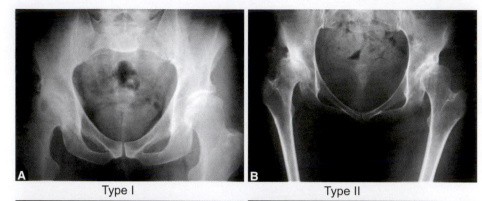

Type I   Type II

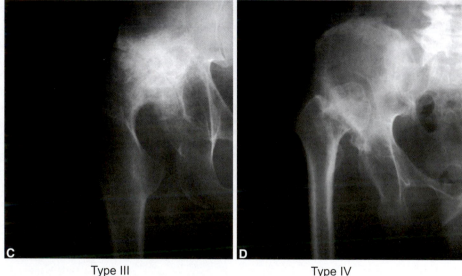

Type III   Type IV

Figures 1A to D: Crowe's grading of dysplasia

socket. Each of these types are further subdivided depending on type of acetabular deficiency.

Dr Thomas Gross from South Carolina has been working extensively on reconstruction of dysplastic hips. He has been propagating the idea that the acetabular socket is oval and not round (personal communication). The challenge therefore in acetabular reconstruction is fitting a hemispherical component into this native oval structure. He is of the opinion that the longitudinal axis of this oval socket is in the posteroinferior to the anterosuperior direction. Thereby most of the acetabular bone stock is preserved in the posterior, inferior and medial aspects. I find this to me a very important principle for the surgeon to be aware of, so that the reaming can start with posterior bias and proceed from posteroinferior to an anterosuperior direction. I also find that the shape of the femoral head is a good clue as to the what one can expect on the acetabular side. If the head is flat then the socket is also very likely to be shallow without any depth (mirror image). A standard cup may be difficult in this situation. I have used, the dysplasia cups (from the Birmingham system) with superior bolts in this situation. In contrast, if the head is circular one can expect a nice deep socket to implant a standard acetabular cup.

SURGICAL INDICATIONS

Surgical intervention in patients with dysplastic hips is indicated when they develop end-stage osteoarthritis with severe hip pain and their activities of daily life (ADL) are compromised. This applies to Crowe's types I, II and III. In bilaterally affected patients with Crowe's type IV dysplasia, surgery is considered only in case of severe pain and not because the patient has a limping gait. As surgery for these hips are often complex, associated with serious complications and result in inferior outcomes when compared to osteoarthritis, surgeons and patients must judiciously evaluate their options before embarking on such procedures.

PREOPERATIVE PREPARATION

A thorough clinical examination to assess the deformity is necessary. This will aid in planning the reconstruction of the hip joint. The degree of pelvic tilt and lumbar lordosis will indicate the compensatory effort to regain balance in the pelvis. These compensatory mechanisms may persist through the postoperative period. It is important to remind the patient to overcome and reverse these mechanisms by physical therapy during post-operative rehabilitation. It is also important to note the limb-length discrepancy clinically. The surgeon must remember to correlate this to the radiological discrepancy. If the limb-length difference is more apparent on the radiograph than clinically, it may indicate compensatory femoral overgrowth on the affected side. In such a situation, the surgeon must not attempt overzealous correction of the limb-length discrepancy. Any previous surgical scars around the hip may indicate surgical intervention at a younger age. Appropriate history must be elicited from the patient in this matter. Extensive or complex interventions may have induced fibrosis around the hip joint converting a previously lax joint into a fibrotic one. Radiographic assessment must include anteroposterior (AP) and lateral views of the afflicted joint. Computed tomographic (CT) scans can aid in assessment of the acetabular bone stock and femoral anteversion, which are difficult to gauge on a plain radiograph. The surgeon must also preorder small sizes of acetabular cup and be prepared to even implant a 22 mm femoral head. It may be necessary to perform a greater trochanter or sub-trochanteric osteotomy, in which case a distal diaphyseal fixation with a modular cementless stem may be essential. Very rarely are acetabular reinforcement rings or bulk acetabular grafts necessary.

SURGICAL CONSIDERATIONS

A standard surgical procedure with standard primary components suffice for majority of the dysplastic hips. For severe deformities or high riding hips, the four key issues that need to be addressed are acetabular hypoplasia, femoral hypoplasia and deformity, restoration of the abductor function and limb-length discrepancy.

Surgical Approach

One may perform the reconstruction either by the anterolateral or posterolateral approaches, though the posterolateral approach is more extensile. In Crowe Type IV hips, if *in situ* implantation of the acetabular cup is planned a trochanteric osteotomy may provide an excellent acetabular exposure. Trochanteric reattachment following completion of the reconstruction will help adjust the abductor tension. On the other hand, if femoral shortening is planned, a sub-trochanteric osteotomy will make exposure of the hip easier. The surgeon can also derotate the femur to correct excessive femoral anteversion. Reconstruction of Crowe type I hips are the most simple. The dysplasia is minimal on both the acetabular and femoral sides, and the surgeon may implant standard implants without any extra effort. Both cemented and uncemented components work well. The difficulty in reconstructing Crowe type II and type III hips arises from the variable loss of the superior acetabular bone stock. In the long-term, uncemented cups fare well in such scenarios.

Acetabular Reconstruction

The areas of concern in reconstructing the dys-plastic acetabulum are placement of the acetabular component close to the anatomic hip center, obtaining maximum host bone coverage of the acetabular component, preserving the native bone stock of the patient as far as possible, obtaining stable primary fixation of the implant, avoiding the use of structural bone graft if possible and medializing the cup to increase femoral offset and optimize the abductor function. The amount of host bone cover over the acetabular component is dependent on the degree of acetabular deficiency and the size of the acetabular component employed. About 70% host bone cover is sufficient for effective stability and fixation of the acetabular component. In the absence of such cover, the surgeon has to employ one of the several techniques listed below:

Medialization

Johnston[3] and Marti[4] reported that loads on the hip were lowered significantly by placing the center of the acetabulum as far medially, inferiorly and anteriorly as anatomically feasible. Linde[5] reported that at an average of 9 years follow-up of cemented Charnley cups, 42% of the cups that were positioned outside the true acetabulum were loose compared to only 13% of cups when placed within the true acetabulum.

Medial Wall Perforation

Dorr[6] advocated the technique of reaming through the acetabular medial wall and placing the acetabular cup on an average of more than 40% beyond the Kohler's line. Twenty four hips with Crowe type II to IV dysplasia had excellent results at 5 to 13 years follow-up. However, this technique sacrifices bone stock from the medial wall and this may compromise later revision procedures. Late migration of the cup into the pelvis is also another possibility.

Medial Wall Displacement Osteotomy

Lian[7] and Yoo[8] described this technique of displacing the acetabular medial wall circumferentially following an osteotomy enabling medial placement of the acetabular component. This allows the surgeon

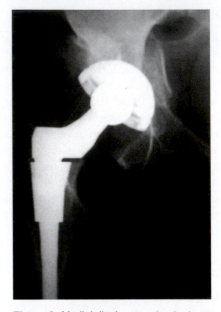

Figure 2: Medial displacement osteotomy

to achieve an optimal hip center of rotation, maximal host bone cover and permits the use of a large acetabular component. Medial bone stock is preserved to simplify future revision procedures (Figure 2).

However, a distinct disadvantage of medialization is that the cup size is limited by the AP diameter of the native acetabulum.[9] Medialization also risks posterior and inferior impingement, thus the surgeon must ensure sufficient femoral offset.

Small Cup with Screw Fixation

In the patient with Crowe type IV dysplasia with a high riding dislocation, the true acetabulum is usually very small and shallow. The acetabular fossa is thin with very little bone stock. Due to this limitation, reconstruction with an extra small cementless cup and multiple screw fixation must be considered. A 22 mm femoral head is preferred to increase the poly liner thickness. Hampton et al. have reported an average 16 year survival of 92% with the use of a hemispherical porous-coated acetabular component in twenty consecutive total hip replacements in severe developmental dysplasia of the hips (Figures 3A and B).

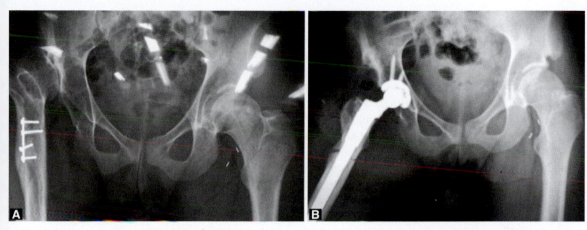

Figures 3A and B: Small cup with high hip center and subtrochanteric osteotomy

Roof Reconstruction

Augmenting the superolateral deficiency of the acetabulum with bone graft may be helpful.[10] This may be resorted to when more than 30% of the cup is uncovered. A rule of thumb that I often apply is to rely on the shape of the femoral head on the pre-operative radiograph of the pelvis. If the femoral head is round, then it is most likely to be contained and would not require supplemental fixation. On the other hand if the femoral head is non-spherical or "mushroom-shaped", then it is more likely not to be contained in the acetabular cavity, and such a reconstruction would in all probability require supplemental fixation in the form of screws or even autografts from the femoral head. Graft stability and fixation is superior with corticocancellous bone when compared to cancellous chip grafts. Use of cement to augment at this region is clearly inferior to bone graft. Autografts from the patient's own femoral head is superior to using allografts. Lastly, the structural grafts can provide additional bone stock to facilitate subsequent revision surgery. It is important to remember that one cannot rely on the graft to be load-bearing. In other words, the graft must be in addition to the primary stability of the cup. The surgeon must not rely on the graft to provide stability in the absence of primary cup fixation. Bone augmentation in this manner has limited application as large structural grafts tend to fail with high load

situations. Mulroy[11] has reported 50% failure at 12 years with major structural bone grafts. Graft failures were also higher when the acetabular component was implanted 1 cm higher than its anatomical center.[12]

Acetabular Reinforcement Ring

These devices allow the load to bypass the structural graft thus protecting it from resorption and collapse. Even when resorption occurs, the reinforcement ring protects the polyethylene cup from being directly affected.[13] Zehntner[14] has reported satisfactory mid-term results with this technique.

Double or Oblong Acetabular Prostheses

These devices can also be utilized to cover large deficient areas of the acetabulum, however they have not been in popular practice.[15,16]

High Hip Center

Harris[17] was the first to describe the high hip center for acetabular reconstruction in acetabuli with significant bone loss. Studies have demonstrated that biomechanically a high hip center without lateralization does not affect the prosthetic hip. There are several advantages to this technique. The surgeon does not have to resort to bringing the femur down as often this is risky and difficult to achieve.

Quality of bone at the false acetabulum is generally good as the femoral head has been articulating at this region for a long time. For the same reason, often bone grafting is not required at this level. Most often a small acetabular component has to be used at this nonanatomical region. Issues with this technique are that the leg-length discrepancy remains under corrected, postoperative limping persists and often there is no option but to position the cup laterally leading to poor abductor function. The surgeon must make a note to check for impingement with the anteriorsuperior iliac spine during flexion and with the ischial tuberosity in extension. Reports on the high hip center are conflicting in the literature at the moment. Callaghan[18] has reported high risk of loosening with a high hip center when compared to implantation at the anatomic level. Pagano,[19] however found no correlation between the height of the hip center and risk of loosening. In general, it is by and large accepted that acetabular component placement at the anatomic level yields better outcomes. But in situations of dysplastic hips where the bone stock at the anatomic level is inadequate and large structural bone grafts may be required, it would be prudent to implant the component at a higher level. It is important to recognize that in case of placing the component at a higher level, medializing the cup is critical to avoid the stresses associated with lateral placement of the acetabular component.

Femoral Reconstruction (Figures 4A and B)

Femoral reconstruction is simpler compared to the acetabular side in dysplasia. In Crowe type I and II hips, the femur differs very little from the normal and can generally accept a standard primary stem component. In such cases, the femur is slightly hypoplastic with a valgus neck angle and excessive anteversion. In Crowe types III and IV, the femoral intramedullary canal is narrow, with a posteriorly displaced greater trochanter and increased limb-length discrepancy. Longitudinal osteotomy may be required to accommodate the femoral component.

Limb-length restoration is a greater challenge on the femoral side. With a high hip center this may not be an issue, otherwise this often implies some type

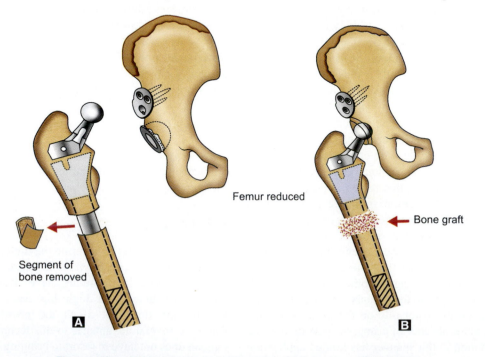

Femur reduced

Bone graft

Segment of bone removed

A

B

Figures 4A and B: Subtrochanteric osteotomy. (A) Osteotomy; (B) Reduction of osteotomy on the proximal femur. The degree of limb lengthening that can be achieved without resorting to an osteotomy is limited by tension on the sciatic nerve. If the sciatic nerve is tight, which can be often assessed by palpation, then the surgeon must not hesitate to perform an osteotomy. There are two principal osteotomies in the proximal femur. One is to perform a trochanteric osteotomy,[20,21] resect the proximal femur and then re-attach the trochanter to the femoral shaft, preferably more anteriorly. As the metaphysis is sacrificed, standard uncemented stems will not suffice. Nonunion of the trochanter can also be an issue as the trochanter is abutting against cortical bone. The second method is to perform a subtrochanteric shortening osteotomy.[22-25]

This method preserves the proximal femur with its muscle attachments making the hip more stable. The femur can also be derotated to account for the excess anteversion of the femur. Oblique, step-cuts and transverse cuts have been advocated at the osteotomy site. The modularity of the S-ROM stem confers significant benefits, as the proximal femur can be prepared separately to achieve a good purchase by the proximal sleeve (Figure 5).

The distal femur can then be independently prepared to receive the distal end of the stem. Unless

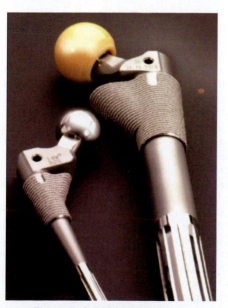

Figure 5: S-ROM femoral stems

I have performed the osteotomy for better exposure of the hip joint, I plan the osteotomy following the acetabular component implantation. After sizing the S-ROM stem, I implant the definitive proximal sleeve. Keeping a trial sleeve outside the bone to identify the distal extent of the definitive sleeve I score the femoral shaft about an 1-1.5 cm distally to mark the level of the osteotomy and a longitudinal reference line perpendicular to it. The longitudinal reference line helps to match the proximal and distal ends of the osteotomied femur during stem insertion. Following this I perform the osteotomy in an transverse fashion across the femur. With the proximal end, I proceed to prepare the placement of the sleeve, and attempt reduction of the head into the acetabular socket. At this point, the proximal end of the femur tends to over-ride the distal end of the femur. This point is again scored on the femur, and I proceed with a second osteotomy on the distal femur. Once this is complete, I proceed with preparation of the distal femur. Many times the osteotomy ends will not be a perfect match and will oppose one another in oblique fashion. The oblique orientation can be corrected by nibbling one end till the osteotomized ends achieve a snap fit. Thus, it is important to under resect the segment. Masonis[26] reported the successful use of the S-ROM stem with shortening osteotomy for femoral reconstruction in dysplastic hips achieving excellent pain relief and improvement in hip function. They reported no failures in their series of dysplastic hips.

COMPLICATIONS

Common complications observed with such complex reconstructions are sciatic nerve palsy, dislocation in the postoperative period, high wear situation and early failure, increased infection rate, trochanteric and subtrochanteric nonunion, intraoperative acetabular fracture and component protrusio, and intraoperative femoral fracture.

SUMMARY

Reconstruction of the dysplastic hip is a complex procedure fraught with potential complications.

The main issue is acetabular dysplasia. Achieving rigid primary fixation with uncemented acetabular components with adequate host bone contact is critical for good long-term results. As far as possible the cup must be implanted close to the normal anatomical hip center, and the use of larger structural bone grafts must be avoided. Subtrochanteric osteotomy is a safe procedure to contend with to bring the femoral head to achieve a stable functional articulating fit with the acetabular socket.

REFERENCES

1. Crowe JF, Mani VJ, Ranawat CS. Total hip replacement in congenital dislocation and dysplasia of the hip. J Bone Joint Surg Am 1979;61:15-23.
2. Hartofilakidis G, Stamos K, Karachalios T, Ioannidis TT, Zacharakis N. Congenital hip disease in adults—classification of acetabular deficiencies and operative treatment with acetabuloplasty combined with total hip arthroplasty. J Bone Joint Surg Am 1996;78:683-92.
3. Johnston RC, Brand RA, Crowninshield RD. Reconstruction of the hip—a mathematical approach to determine optimum geometric relationships. J Bone Joint Surg Am 1979;61:639-52.
4. Marti RK, Schuller HM, van Steijn MJ. Supero-lateral bone grafting for acetabular deficiency in primary total hip replacement and revision. J Bone Joint Surg Br 1994;76:728-34.
5. Linde F, Jensen J, Pilgaard S. Charnley arthroplasty in osteoarthritis secondary to congenital dislocation or subluxation of the hip. Clin Orthop Relat Res 1988;227:164-71.
6. Dorr LD, Tawakkol S, Moorthy M, Long W, Wan Z. Medial protrusio technique for placement of a porous-coated, hemispherical acetabular component without cement in a total hip arthroplasty in patients who have acetabular dysplasia. J Bone Joint Surg Am 1999;81:83-92.
7. Lian YY, Yoo MC, Pei FX, Cho YJ, Cheng JQ, et al. Circumferential osteotomy of the medial acetabular wall in total hip replacement for the late sequelae of childhood septic arthritis of the hip. J Bone Joint Surg Br 2007;89:1149-54. doi: 10.1302/0301-620X.89B9.18908. URLhttp://dx.doi.org/10.1302/0301-620X.89B9.18908.
8. Yoo MC, Cho YJ, Kim Kl, Rhyu KH, Chun YS, et al. Cementless total hip arthroplasty with medial wall osteotomy for the sequelae of septic arthritis of the hip. Clin Orthop Surg 2009;1:19-26. doi:10.4055/cios.2009.1.1.19. URLhttp://dx.doi.org/10.4055/cios. 2009.1.1.19.
9. Schuller HM, Dalstra M, Huiskes R, Marti RK. Total hip reconstruction in acetabular dysplasia—a finite element study. J Bone Joint Surg Br 1993;75:468-74.
10. de Jong PT, Haverkamp D, van der Vis HM, Marti RK. Total hip replacement with a superolateral bone graft for osteoarthritis secondary to dysplasia: a long-term follow-up. J Bone Joint Surg Br 2006;88:173-178. doi:10.1302/030i-620X.88B2.16769. URLhttp://dx.doi.org/10.1302/0301-620X.88B2.16769.
11. Mulroy RD, Harris WH. Failure of acetabular autogenous grafts in total hip arthro-plasty. increasing incidence: a follow-up note. J Bone Joint Surg Am 1990;72:1536-40.
12. Atilla B, Ali H, Aksoy MC, Caglar O, Tokgozoglu AM, et al. Position of the acetabular component determines the fate of femoral head autografts in total hip replacement for acetabular dysplasia. J Bone Joint Surg Br 2007;89:874-78. doi:10.1302/0301-620X.89B7.18417. URL http://dx.doi.org/10.1302/0301-620X.89B7.18417.
13. Gill TJ, Sledge JB, Muller ME. Total hip arthroplasty with use of an acetabular reinforcement ring in patients who have congenital dysplasia of the hip. results at five to fifteen years. J Bone Joint Surg Am 1998;80:969-79.
14. Zehntner MK, Ganz R. Midterm results (5.5-10 years) of acetabular allograft reconstruction with the acetabular reinforcement ring during total hip revision. J Arthroplasty 1994;9:469-79.
15. Fousek J, Vasek P. Oblong cup in the management of aseptic loosening of the acetabular component in total hip replacement. Scand J Surg 2007;96:319-24.
16. Berry DJ, Sutherland CJ, Trousdale RT, Colwell CW, Chandler HP, et al. Bilobed oblong porous coated acetabular components in revision total hip arthroplasty. Clin Orthop Relat Res 2000. pp.154-60.
17. Harris WH, Crothers O, Oh I Total hip replacement and femoral-head bone-grafting for severe acetabular deficiency in aduits. J Bone Joint Surg Am 1977;59:752-9.
18. Callaghan JJ, Salvati EA, Pellicci PM, Wilson PD, Ranawat CS. Results of revision for mechanical failure after cemented total hip replacement, 1979 to 1982—a two to five-year follow-up. J Bone Joint Surg Am 1985;67:1074-85.
19. Pagnano W, Hanssen AD, Lewallen DG, Shaughnessy WJ. The effect of superior placement

of the acetabular component on the rate of loosening after total hip arthroplasty. J Bone Joint Surg Am 1996;78:1004-14.

20. Numair J, Joshi AB, Murphy X, Porter ML, Hardinge K. Total hip arthroplasty for congenital dysplasia or dislocation of the hip. survivorship analysis and long-term results. J Bone Joint Surg Am 1997;79:1352-60.

21. Benum P. Transposition of the apophysis of the greater trochanter for reconstruction of the femoral head after septic hip arthritis in children. Acta Orthop 2011;82:64-8. doi:10.3109/17453674.2010.548030.URLhttp://dx.doi.org/10.3109/17453674.2010. 548030.

22. Sponseller PD, McBeath AA (1988) Subtrochanterio osteotomy with intramedullary fixation for arthroplasty of the dysplastio hip—a case report. J Arthroplasty 1988;3:351-54.

23. Akiyama H, Kawanabe K, Yamamoto K, Kuroda Y, So K, et al. Cemented total hip arthroplasty with subtrochanteric femoral shortening transverse osteotomy for severely dislocated hips—outcome with a 3- to 10-year follow-up period. J Orthop Sci 2011;16:270-7. doi:10.1007/s00776-011-0049-z. URLhttp://dx. doi.org/10.1007/ s00776-011-0049-z.

24. Takao M, Ohzono K, Nishii T, Miki H, Nakamura N, et al. Cementless modular total hip arthroplasty with subtrochanteric shortening osteotomy for hips with developmental dysplasia. J Bone Joint Surg Am 2011;93:548-55. doi:10.2106/JBJS.I.01619. URL http://dx.dol.Org/10.2106/JBJS.I.01619.

25. Charity JAF, Tsiridis E, Sheeraz A, Howell JR, Hubble MJW, et al. Treatment of crowe IV high hip dysplasia with total hip replacement using the exeter stem and shortening derota-tional subtrochanteric osteotomy. J Bone Joint Surg Br 2011;93:34-8. doi: 10.1302/0301-620X. 93B1.24689. URL http://dx.doi.org/10.1302/0301-620X.93Bl.24689.

26. Masonis JL, Patel JV, Miu A, Bourne RB, McCalden R, et al. Subtrochanteric shortening and derotational osteotomy in primary total hip arthroplasty for patients with severe hip dysplasia: 5-year follow-up. J Arthroplasty 2003;18:68-73, doi:10. 1054/arth.2003.50104. URL http://dx.doi.org/10. 1054/arth.2003.50104.

13 | Hip Arthroplasty in Tumors Around the Hip Joint

Shishir Rastogi, Shah Alam Khan, Ashok Kumar

INTRODUCTION

Till very recently the viable option for malignant tumors around the hip consisted of an amputation with poor mobility and high morbidity of the survivor.[1,2] Remarkable advances in implant technology, surgical reconstructive techniques and adoption of new chemotherapy protocols have provided limb salvage as a realistic option to the treating surgeon.[1,3] Endoprosthetic replacement with implantation of megaprosthesis is a widely accepted alternative in limb salvage surgery for malignant and aggressive lesions in and around the hip joint.

History of Endoprosthetic Use in Bone Tumors

It is interesting to note that the very first hip (hemi) arthroplasty was performed by Moore for a recurrent GCT of the proximal femur.[4] He had used a 25 cm long Vitallium mould for the upper end of the femur. The patient was reported to have active range of motion about three quarters of the normal. The credit for modern endoprosthetic designs goes to Kenneth Francis and Ralph Marcove, who in 1970, described their prosthesis for an osteosarcoma around the knee joint.[5] Early custom-made endoprostheses were prepared based on the radiological extent of the tumor. But they had many disadvantages including 8 to 10 weeks of delay in manufacturing and mismatch in the actual required size of implants either due to incorrect preoperative measurement or change in the extent of the tumor resection and increased complication rates.[6] Introduction of the modular prosthesis in 1980 allowed to avoid the

problems of custom made prosthesis. It also reduced the cost of the implant and was more acceptable due to a relatively low complication rate.

INDICATIONS OF HIP ARTHROPLASTY IN BONE TUMORS

Management of tumors around the hip joint requires a coordinated team effort which should facilitate early diagnosis and definitive management of the lesion in question. The basic aim of performing a hip arthroplasty in a bone tumor around the hip should be to obtain a tumor-free margin (important in malignant lesions), provide stability to the hip construct and thereby increase patient mobility. The indications of hip arthroplasty would therefore be all resectable primary malignant tumors affecting the proximal femur or the acetabulum and metastatic lesions affecting the proximal femur or the acetabulum. The use of arthroplasty in benign tumors of the proximal femur are well documented.[7] These include aggressive (Campanacci Grade III) giant cell tumors, fibro-histiocytomas and extensive and destructive aneurysmal bone cysts involving the articular margins of the proximal femur or the acetabulum.

CONTRAINDICATIONS OF HIP ARTHROPLASTY IN BONE TUMORS

Absolute contraindications of limb salvage surgery with hip replacement include tumors with more than one compartment involvement, patients with

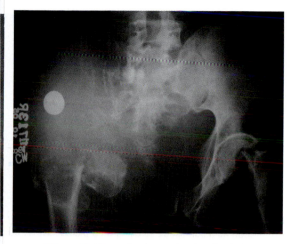

Figure 1: Excessive tumor load—absolute contraindication to surgery

healing capacities thereby posing special risks in the postoperative period. Finally, there are differences in rehabilitation schedules and satisfaction levels in patients undergoing limb salvage surgery for tumors around the hip as compared to those undergoing a primary THR.

PREOPERATIVE EVALUATION

Special surgeries require special work-ups. A thorough clinical and radiological work-up of a lesion around the hip is essential before deciding on any surgery in the area. The evaluation should aim to establish the diagnosis, stage the lesion and give an insight into the planning of the expected surgery so as to obtain optimum functional results.

an expected life span of less than six weeks, tumors of the proximal femur, which cannot be resected without excising the important muscles, e.g., the hip abductors, that are tumors with excessive tumor volume (Figure 1). Involvement of the femoral neurovascular bundle is now considered as a relative contraindication to salvage since newer promising methods of bypass and repair are now available. Infection in a tumor is an absolute contraindication to salvage. It is also important to stress that a lack of surgical know-how in musculoskeletal oncology should be considered as a contraindication to surgery.

1. Clinical evaluation of the patient is essential in establishing a diagnosis and planning treatment. The main aim of the clinical examination for primary tumors around the hip joint should be to examine the size, size and multiplicity of the swelling. The clinical examination should be able to assess the local skin condition and the involvement of the neurovascular bundle. Huge pelvic filling tumors can be difficult to examine as the underlying structures are stretched taut by the underlying mass (Figure 2).

Tumors around the hip are known to present late as the initial clinical features are masked since the pain causing structures lie deep under a dense cover of muscles. Emphasis should be made to assess the efficiency and involvement of

HOW IS HIP ARTHROPLASTY IN BONE TUMORS DIFFERENT FROM A PRIMARY REPLACEMENT?

Hip arthroplasty in bone tumors around the hip joint is a special surgery, remarkably different from a primary Total hip replacement (THR). The procedure is different in more than one way. It requires special, customized implants, which are different from the less constrained implants used in a conventional THR. The surgical technique is special as there is non-availability of normal musculature around the hip joint. The anatomical landmarks are poorly defined, requiring clinical acumen to judge the surgical margins. It is also important to note that patients with malignant disease who undergo neoadjuvant chemotherapy prior to a salvage surgery have poor

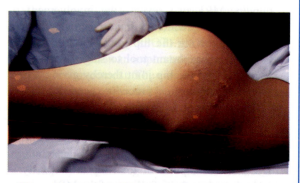

Figure 2: A massive ABC of the proximal femur difficult to examine huge lesions

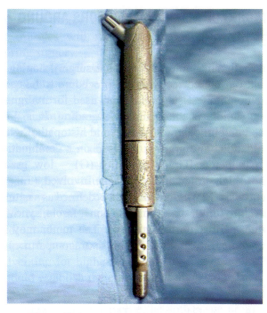

Figure 7: A conventional hip endoprosthesis (without the head)

fenestrations on its lateral ridge (trochanter part) for attaching the abductors and external rotators.

2. *Head:* Usually a bipolar head for host acetabulum, it comes in standard sizes (38-56 mm) with variable neck lengths (+5 , 0, –5).

3. *Stem:* Different sizes (diameters: 9-13 mm) are available, it should have minimal 9-10 mm intramedullary length and round proximal portion should rest on the bone at the site bone osteotomy and it may articulate directly with articular segment or with the extension piece proximally.

4. *Resection piece/extension piece/spacers:* These come in different sizes (length: 35-95 mm), it articulates with the stem distally and with articular segment proximally.

Total length is usually around 135-200 cm, diameter is 14-18 mm, has a anterior bow, has extramedullary porous in growth material on the segment proximal to stem.

SURGICAL TECHNIQUE

Endoprosthesis allows intraoperative flexibility for reconstruction of the long segmental defect, immediate stability, early rehabilitation, immediate weight-bearing is durable and gives better functional outcome than arthrodesis.[15]

Surgical Technique of Endoprosthesis

A good surgical technique requires meticulous planning. The limb should be drapped with the distal limb and the knee joint exposed (Figure 8).

The Smith-Peterson anterior approach is the preferred approach for resection of all tumors of the proximal femur. Large tumors with huge soft tissue component need meticulous dissection for separating the surrounding neurovascular bundle from the tumor. Anterior approach allows dissection of the neurovascular bundle under direct supervision. In tumors with both an anterior and a posterior component, an extensile approach is used.

Skin incision is given starting 5 cm proximal to anterior superior iliac spine along the iliac blade and then extending vertically down into the thigh up to 5 cm distal to proposed osteotomy site for resection of bone tumor. Plane is developed between the rectus femoris and the tensor fascia lata proximally and between Sartorius and rectus femoris distally. In the upper part of the incision femoral neurovascular structures are identified and depending upon the proximal extent of the tumor inguinal ligament may also be incised to get the control over the external iliac vessels in proximally advanced tumor. Plane is developed along the medial and proximal

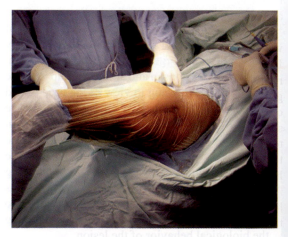

Figure 8: The limb should be drapped with the knee joint free

margins of tumor by gentle blunt dissection using the small artery forceps. Peanuts made of rolled small gauze piece on artery forceps are used to separate the neurovascular bundles from the tumor by gentle dissection. Neurovascular bundles should be separated throughout the length from the tumor under direct supervision. Stay sutures are applied in the capsule and is incised along the neck of the femur; head is dislocated by flexion adduction and internal rotation after cutting the ligamentum teres. Careful attention is given to the abductors involvement; a bony sleeve should be separated with the abductors if trochanter is spared. If trochanter is also involved then abductors and external rotators (1cm enbloc) are cut from the trochanter after putting stay sutures. Proximally adductors, flexors are cut from the femur having a visibly tumor free end after putting stay sutures (Figure 9).

Next the length of the femoral resection is measured from the head to the distal tumor margin determined by preoperative MRI and on table by visualization of the tumor (Figure 10).

Osteotomy is usually done distal (3-4 cm for primary sarcoma and 1-2 cm for metastasis) to this measured length of resection. Medullary curettes are taken from the distal end of the osteotomy (normal bone and not from the distal end of tumor) and are sent for examination of tumor cells on a frozen section. Frozen sections can also be sent from the cotyloid cavity on suspicion of its involvement. Next the remaining muscles are removed from the linea aspera and the tumor is removed (Figure 11).

Hemostasis is achieved, the wound packed and we wait for the result of the frozen study. Once the frozen is confirmed to be negative for tumor tissue, reaming is started with an 8 or 9 mm reamer and gradually increased up to the maximum diameter chosen for the canal. Definitive intramedullary stem should be 1-2 mm less than the size of last reamer to accommodate the cement. Now assembly of the endoprosthesis is started according to the total length of the resected proximal femoral segment. Articular segment is attached with the desired length of extension pieces which are attached to the intramedullary stem by impaction using the impaction platform. Next this piece is used as a trial

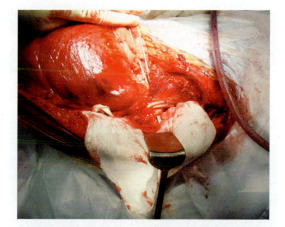

Figure 9: Proximally abductors and rotators are being separated

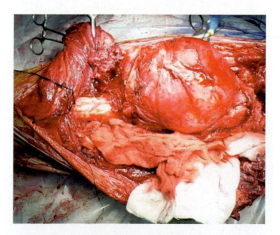

Figure 10: Tumor separated distally and proximally

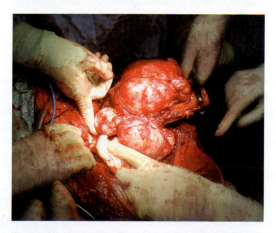

Figure 11: Tumor freed from proximal and distal sides

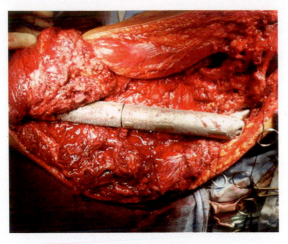

Figure 12: Showing the prosthesis *in situ* (without the head)

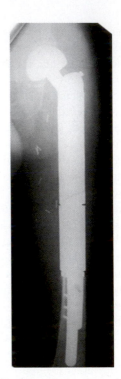

Figure 14: Postoperative radiograph of a patient with an HMRS endoprosthesis

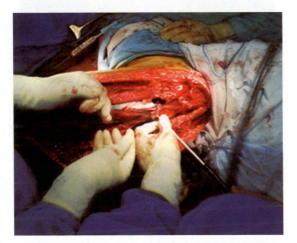

Figure 13: Abductors and external rotators are being attached to trochanteric part of the prosthesis

by inserting the intramedullary stem and attaching the trial bipolar head to check the length, stability and version. A mark by cautery or gentian violet is made on the anterior midpoint and on the linea aspera to insert the stem in correct version and correct position of the trochanteric part (lateral) of the articular segment without cement (Figure 12).

The assembled prosthesis with definitive head is inserted after cementing of the medullary canal using cement gun. Prosthesis is adjusted with 10-15 degrees of anteversion and lateral position of the trochanteric part of articular segment. Once the cement has set, reduction is done and stability is checked.

It is essential to carry out a good and strong soft tissue repair and reconstruction around the prosthesis head. This is important as it gives stability to an otherwise unsupported prosthetic head. The capsule is sutured and the abductors, external rotators are tied to the trochanteric part of prosthesis with Ethibond sutures directly or indirectly through a mesh (our technique) sutured around the trochanteric part. Alternatively, the remaining capsule can be brought over the head and neck of the prosthesis and reinforced by circumferential Dacron tape to the vastus lateralis muscle to give immediate stability (Figure 13).

The capsule is then reinforced by tenodesing the pectineus and psoas muscles to the anterior capsule and the external rotators to the posterior capsule. The abductors are then advanced to the prosthesis with Dacron tape and tenodesed. It is a good practice to try and cover the prosthesis by mobilizing the remaining parts of the abductors and vastus lateralis over the prosthesis. Deep fascia is sutured and wound is closed in layer after putting the drain. Dressing is applied.

POSTOPERATIVE PROTOCOL

The wound inspection is done on the 2nd day and sutures removed on 14th day. Partial weight bearing is allowed after the third week, giving time for soft tissue healing. Full weight-bearing is allowed over next 7-10 days depending upon the abductor strength and pain tolerance. Postoperative chemotherapy is started at 4 weeks after the surgery and patient is followed up regularly. Radiographs are taken at regular intervals (Figure 14).

COMPLICATIONS OF THE ENDOPROSTHESIS

Endoprosthetic replacement for a tumor around the hip joint is a complex procedure and is accompanied by its own share of complications. Common complications include delayed healing, wound infection (1-15%; superficial and deep), instability, dislocation, periprosthetic fractures, aseptic loosening (up to 46%) and implant breakage. High incidence of infection is due to extensive soft tissue dissection, long surgery, large dead space, inadequate soft tissue coverage of the prosthesis and immunosuppression due to chemotherapy.[19]

Dislocation is seen in 2-14% of the patients, studies have shown that preservation of the acetabulum and capsule, adequate capsulorrhaphy, proper version and proper abductor reattachment reduces the dislocation rate. Revisions are common and the longevity of the endoprosthesis have been reported 73% at 5 years and around 60-63% at 10 years. Bickels reported a 7.7% revision rate in 39 proximal femoral endoprosthetic reconstruction at a mean follow-up of 80 months.[20] Menendez reported a 3.2% revision rate in 62 at mean follow-up of 18 months. Finstein reported 19.4% revision rate at a mean of 59.2 month's follow-up in a cohort of 62 bipolar reconstructions.[21]

REFERENCES

1. Radoslav Barjaktarović, Zoran Popović, Dragan Radoičić. Megaendoprosthesis in the treatment of bone tumors in the knee and hip region. Strana 62 Vojnosanitetski Pregled. Volumen 68, Broj 1: 62-8
2. Lange B, Kramer S, Gregg J, Toledano S, Wimmer R, Evans A. High-dose methotrexate and Adriamycin in osteogenic sarcoma: The Children's Hospital of Philadelphia Study. Am J Clin Oncol. 1982;5:3-8.
3. Bernthal NM, Schwartz AJ, Oakes DA, Kabo JM, Eckardt JJ. How long do endoprosthetic reconstructions for proximal femoral tumors last? . Clin Orthop Relat Res. 2010;468(11):2867-74.
4. Moore AT, Bohlman HR. Metal hip joint: a case report. J Bone Joint Surg 1943;25:688-92.
5. Marcove RC, Lewis MM, Rosen G, et al. Total femur and total knee replacement. A preliminary report. Clin Orthop 1977;126:147-52.
6. Robert Henshaw, Martin Malawer. Review of Endoprosthetic Reconstruction in Limb-sparing Surgery. In: Martin M Malawer, Paul H Sugarbaker (Eds). Musculoskeletal Cancer Surgery Treatment of Sarcomas and Allied Diseases. Kluwer Academic Publishers; 2001. pp.381-402.
7. Khan SA, Kumar A, Inna P, Bakhshi S, Rastogi S. Endoprosthetic replacement for giant cell tumour of proximal femur. J of Orthopaedic Surg 2009;17(3): 280-3.
8. Adler LP, Blair HF, Makley JT, et al. Comparison of PET with CT, MRI, and conventional scintigraphy in a benign and in a malignant soft tissue tumor. Orthopedics 1991;14:891.
9. Jaffe HL. Introduction: Problems of classification and diagnosis. In: Jaffe HL, (Ed). Tumors and Tumorous Conditions of the Bones and Joints. Philadelphia: Lea and Febiger; 1958.pp.9-17.
10. Enneking WF, Spanier SS, Goodman MA. A system for the surgical staging of musculoskeletal sarcoma. Clin Orthop Relat Res 1980;153:106.
11. Bramwell, Bramwell VHC. The role of chemotherapy in osteogenic sarcoma. Crit Rev Oncol Hematol 1995;20:61.
12. Ferguson WS, Goorin AM. Current treatment of osteosarcoma. Cancer Invest 2001;19(3):292-315.
13. Blay JY, Bouhour D, Ray-Coquard I, et al. High-dose chemotherapy with autologous hematopoietic stem-cell transplantation for advanced soft tissue sarcoma in adults. J Clin Oncol 2000;18:3643.

14. Grimer RJ, Carter SR, Pynsent PB. The cost-effectiveness of limbsalvage for bone tumours. J Bone Joint Surg Br 1997;79:558-61.

15. Grimer RJ, Carter SR, Tillman RM, Abudu A. Postoperative infection and increased survival in osteosarcoma patients: are they associated? Ann Surg Oncol 2007;14:2887-95.

16. Unwin PS, Cannon SR, Grimer RJ, et al. Aseptic loosening in cemented custom-made prosthetic replacements for bone tumours of the lower limb. J Bone Joint Surg 1996;78-B:5-13.

17. Damron TA. Endoprosthetic replacement following limb-sparing resection for bone sarcoma. Semin Surg Oncol 1997;13:3-10.

18. Jeys LM, Grimer RJ, Carter SR, Tillman RM. Periprosthetic infection in patients treated for an orthopaedic oncological condition. J Bone Joint Surg Am 2005;87(4):842-9.

19. Bickels J, Meller I, Henshaw RM, Malawar MM. Reconstruction of hip stability after proximal and total femur resections. Clin Orthop Relat Res 2000;375:218-30. doi: 10.1097/00003086-200006000-00027.

20. Menendez LR, Ahlmann ER, Kermani C, Gotha H. Endoprosthetic reconstructions for neoplasms of the proximal femur. Clin Orthop Relat Res. 2006;450:46-51. doi: 10.1097/01.blo.0000229332.91158.05.

21. Finstein J, King J, Fox E, Ogilvie C, Lackman R. Bipolar proximal femoral replacement prostheses for musculoskeletal neoplasms. Clin Orthop Relat Res. 2007;459:66-75. doi: 10.1097/BLO.0b013e31804f5474.

14 | Total Hip Arthroplasty in Proximal Femoral Deformity

Rajesh Malhotra

A complex primary total hip arthroplasty is defined as the surgery in which the likelihood of intraoperative technical difficulties, perioperative complications or premature failure is greater than usual. A proximal femoral deformity makes total hip arthroplasty (THA) technically complex and presents specific challenges during surgery to the surgeon trying to create a durable construct and an anatomically accurate reconstruction. The technical considerations may be due to the femoral considerations such as relationship between the femoral prosthesis and the recipient femur (intra-osseous) or due to the altered spatial relationship between the acetabulum and the proximal femur (extraosseous).

ETIOLOGY

The proximal femur may be misshapen or deformed due to a variety of conditions which can be congenital, developmental or acquired.[1-5] The most common condition leading to the misshapen proximal femur is the developmental dysplasia of the hip (DDH). Malunited proximal femoral fractures, prior proximal femoral osteotomies (varus, valgus, McMurray, Schanz osteotomy), childhood septic arthritis especially with pathological fractures, metabolic disorders such as osteomalacia and rickets, fibrous dysplasia, spondyloepiphyseal dysplasias, secondary osteoarthritis (due to Legg-Calve-Perthes' disease, slipped capital femoral epiphysis, etc.) and Paget's disease (with repeated stress fractures and Shepherd Crook deformity) are the other usual causes of such deformities. The femoral canal may be misshapen or either too narrow (e.g. Juvenile rheumatoid arthritis, achondroplastic dwarfism and spondyloepiphyseal dysplasia) or too large (e.g. Rheumatoid arthritis, ankylosing spondylitis) leading to a mismatch between the metaphysis of the proximal femur and the diaphysis.

PATHOANATOMY

There may be significant disturbance of proximal femoral anatomy in the face of deformity locally. The deformity may be torsional, angular and translational in nature or there may be disproportion in the size of the femoral anatomy. There may be significant abnormalities of the greater and lesser trochanters and metaphysis (Figure 1). The proximal

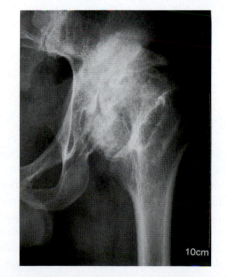

Figure 1: Severely deformed proximal femur showing abnormality of trochanters and metaphysis

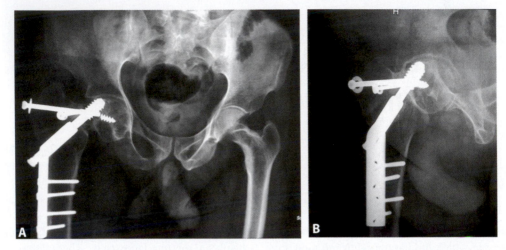

Figures 2A and B: Presence of implants *in situ* presents special problems such as bone remodeling around the implant, formation of neocortex and stress risers in the bone after removal

fragment may be angulated in the frontal plane, in excessive valgus or varus, or in the lateral plane in ante- or retroversion. The proximal fragment is often translated in relation to distal fragment leading to off-ending of the canal in the two fragments. Significant limb length shortening is common. When a medial displacement osteotomy is performed, a spike of the proximal medial femoral cortex will occupy the metaphysis and interfere with canal preparation. There may be remodeling changes in the surrounding bone especially in the presence of internal fixation devices. Neocortex may form around the implant and the canal may be obliterated (Figures 2A and B). Malunion or nonunion of trochanters may be present. Infection may exist in case of a previous surgery especially with implantation of hardware.

PREOPERATIVE PLANNING

The history of a previous surgical intervention and the presence of previous implants from such prior hip surgery are quite relevant in preoperative planning. One must try to determine the type of implants, the manufacturer and the surgical approach chosen for implantation. The presence of screw holes, channels, bone remodeling, broken hardware, or well-osseointegrated piece of hardware will influence surgical approach and implant selection for THA. Presence of sclerotic bone in the medullary

canal at the site of osteotomy or previous fracture may misguide drill bits or rasps and lead to femoral canal perforation. Special attention should be given to assess abductor lever arm and femoral offset to restore abductor power and approximate anatomy. Consideration must be given to how the correction of deformity will affect knee alignment and leg length.

Clinical examination must determine hip mobility and identify muscle contractures and weaknesses. Furthermore, localization of previous skin incisions, skin quality and subcutaneous soft tissue coverage over the greater trochanter or hardware is of paramount importance. Special attention should be paid to leg lengths and neurovascular status.

Radiological examination must evaluate the full extent of the deformity as well as its effect on the mechanical axis of the affected lower limb. Standing films, including the hip, the knee and the ankle allow proper measurement of the mechanical axis and overall alignment of the limb. Anteroposterior and lateral radiographs reveal the site and extent of deformity in the two planes. If malrotation is suspected, an axial computed tomography scan is required, with assessment of difference in orientation between the epicondylar axis at the knee and the femoral neck axis at the hip.[6]

Radiographs also help in identification of equipment and prosthetic need as well as need for a bone graft or osteotomy.

CHALLENGES

The underlying cause of the proximal femoral deformity may lead to distortion of anatomy, alteration of bone quality or both. Standard "off the shelf" implants and routine operative techniques may not allow satisfactory component fit and restoration of both the leg length and the offset. Nonconventional implants and/or techniques are frequently required to optimize intra- and extraosseous relationships. Often there may be soft tissue abnormalities around the hip that must be addressed during reconstruction. The proximal femoral deformity may be a manifestation of a more generalized condition comprising additional orthopedic or medical comorbidities that must be considered during the perioperative period.

Specific Challenges

1. Limb length discrepancy may be coexistent and need equalization.
2. Accurate templating may be difficult. Lateral radiographs may show abnormal angulation of the femoral neck in excessive anteversion or retroversion
3. Risk of lurking infection must be considered in previously operated cases.
4. THA performed after previous procedures are known to present difficulty at exposure.[3]
5. Increased blood loss while dissecting through old scar tissue.
6. Removal of internal fixation devices may be required which may have been *in situ* for decades. This leads to longer surgical time.
7. Poor bone quality due to preexisting osteoporosis.
8. Fractures may occur due to stress concentration from a rasp or femoral component as a result of holes left by the metal implants.[7,8] Also, all the stress risers must be by-passed and that may require use of a long stem/strut allografts thus increasing complexity.
9. Access to canal may be denied by overhanging greater trochanter or obliteration of medullary canal by new bone formation.
10. Greater trochanter disruption, which can lead to increased rate of dislocation and difficult ambulatory function.
11. Implant selection may be challenging in the face of distorted anatomy and bone defects. If a cementless fixation is chosen, it may be difficult to obtain an acceptable fit using a standard implant. Options include a corrective osteotomy or a custom or modular component. When a corrective osteotomy is chosen, a straight stemmed design may be desirable and the presence of distal flutes or splines to enhance rotational stability may be useful. An alternative is extensively porous coated straight stemmed implants available with reduced metaphyseal segments that allow for greater correction of anteversion. Another variant is a "bent rod" without any metaphyseal enlargement. A special double-curved osteotomy stem is useful in certain cases.[3]

    Several currently available designs of modular stems feature metaphyseal segments or sleeves in various sizes to optimize proximal "fit and fill". Such stems (such as S-ROM®, DePuy Orthopaedics Inc, Warsaw, Ind)) may be regarded as off-the-shelf custom implants. Finally, a true custom implant based on three dimensional computed tomography may be employed.[9]

12. With cemented implant, fit may also be problematic. A short cemented stem may be implanted proximal to the deformity. However, small stems with small cement mantles or in suboptimal positions may not provide optimal proximal bone contact or stability. Custom designed femoral prostheses for cemented use may offer a solution.[10]

    Finally, there may be difficulties of cement pressurization in the presence of cortical screw holes.[11]

SURGICAL TECHNIQUE

Treatment must be individualized to address the level of the deformity, type of the deformity, bone quality, and, retained hardware in the proximal femur. Surgeon's experience and preference should also influence the surgical treatment. Surgeon must choose the proper implant and surgical approach and must be familiar with specialized techniques, such as trochanteric osteotomy, corrective osteotomy and limb lengthening.

The various strategies for managing the femoral deformities can be:

1. Osteotomy
   – to alter the bone to fit the prosthesis.[5,12]
2. Modular stem or custom stems
   – to choose a prosthesis to fit the femur.
3. Avoid distal deformity
   – Use surface replacement[13] or short stem.

The level of the deformity also determines the approach to the patient. The deformity of the greater trochanter may not allow proper instrumentation of the femoral canal and osteotomy and advancement of the greater trochanter may be indicated for the proper insertion of the femoral component. The removal of the hardware or the reaming and broaching of the medullary canal are likely to fracture the greater trochanter,[11] and if suspected, it is advisable to perform a controlled osteotomy and advancement of the greater trochanter to avoid the complications of nonunion, malunion, or migration. In case

greater trochanter is ununited or needs osteotomy, it is advisable to keep trochanteric fixation devices, wires, etc. ready.

The deformity at the level of the femoral neck leads to abnormal version and offset. The femoral modular stems which are available in various offsets to establish adequate myofascial tension without affecting limb length are ideally suited for such conditions. The deformity at the metaphysis occurs due to previous trauma or osteotomy. Monobloc metaphyseal filling implants work poorly in this situation due to inadequate fit and increased incidence of fracture. Modular stems work well in this situation.

Metaphyseal/diaphyseal abnormalities lead to mismatch between the metaphysis and diaphysis and again in this situation modular stems allow optimal proximal and distal fit independently. If a subtrochanteric osteotomy has to be performed, then modular stems such as S-ROM can provide rotational stability. Figures 3A to F demonstrate the surgical technique of implantation of S-ROM stem

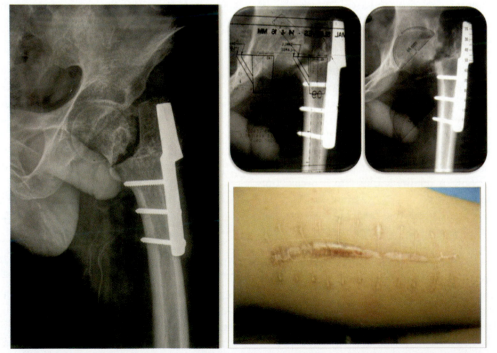

Figure 3A: Secondary osteoarthritis following fracture neck of femur treated with osteotomy fixed with spline. Scar and the preoperative templating for S-ROM are shown

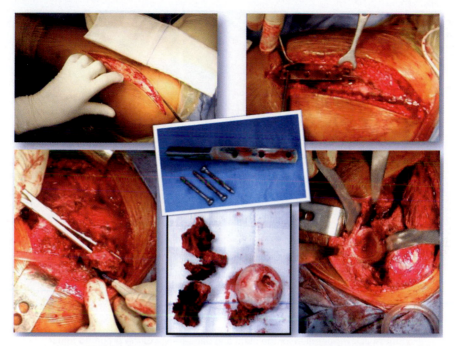

Figure 3B: Removal of implants and the proximal fragment

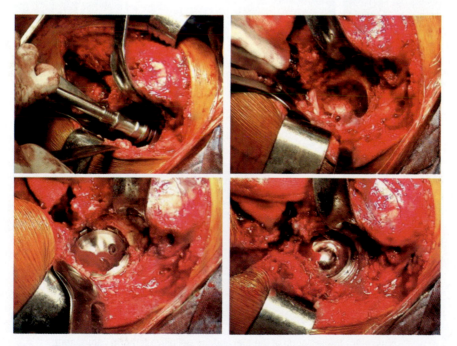

Figure 3C: Preparation of acetabulum and implantation of the component

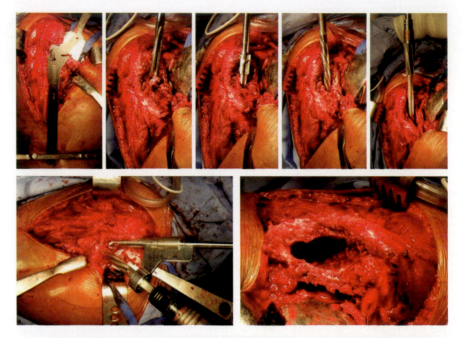

Figure 3D: Preparation for the stem and appearance of the prepared femur

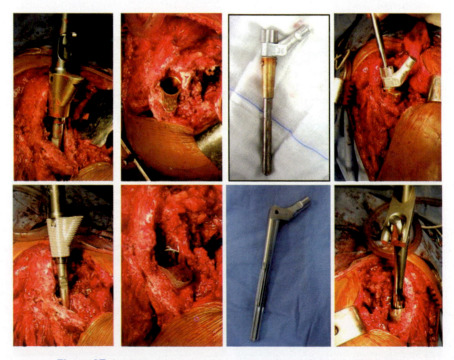

Figure 3E: Implantation of the trial and the definitive femoral component

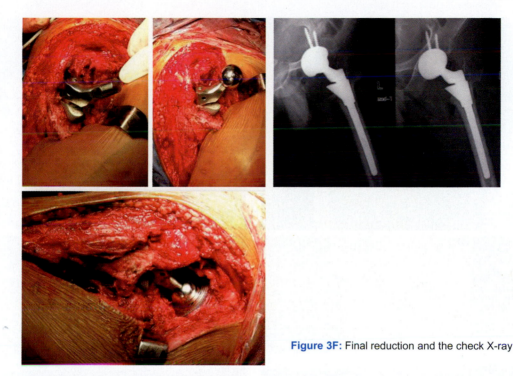

Figure 3F: Final reduction and the check X-ray

for a complex proximal femoral deformity with internal fixation implants *in situ*.

The initial surgical approach is posterior although transtrochanteric approach may be required sometimes where the greater trochanter is overhanging and preventing access to the canal and subtrochanteric osteotomy is otherwise not needed in spite of the deformity. A trochanteric osteotomy may also be required to tension the abductors. Transtrochanteric approach is also useful if the trochanter is ununited from previous trauma or surgery. The femur is provisionally prepared with reaming and broaching. Cementless components circumvent the difficulties of cement escape into the soft tissues and interposition at the osteotomy site. Cylindrical cementless stem designs with features providing distal rotational stability (e.g. extensively coated or fluted designs) are particularly well suited. The neocortex obliterating the canal or the cortical medial spike of the proximal fragment in the canal are not easily penetrated by blunt-tipped intramedullary reamers or broaches, which may be deflected eccentrically. It may be advisable to open the femoral canal with a high-speed burr

before using the standard instrumentation. Figures 4 and 5 illustrate how intramedullary cortical spike can be tackled and modular stem used to achieve a successful reconstruction.

Subtrochanteric osteotomy with or without shortening and/or derotation is applicable to cases of abnormal version[14] or subtrochanteric deformity. Canal preparation after the corrective osteotomy may be facilitated by provisional reduction and fixation of the femur with a plate and clamps.[5] Still it may be very difficult to control the proximal segment. The plate and the clamps should be left in place during the stem impaction in order to prevent distraction of the segments. In all cases with femoral distortion, canal preparation is undertaken cautiously and continued just until initial resistance is met. The broach/reamer is then left in place and biplanar check radiographs are obtained to ensure proper alignment. Endosteal bone deflecting the instrument may need to be removed with a high speed burr to correct malalignment. When preparing the femur for a long stem prosthesis, check films reduce the risk of distal perforation. Following corrective osteotomy, the proximal fragment must be rigidly fixed to the

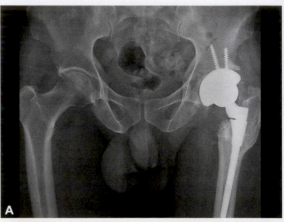

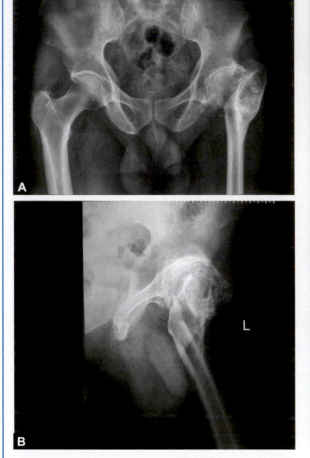

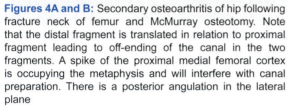

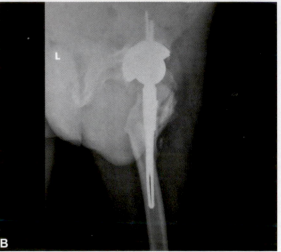

Figures 4A and B: Secondary osteoarthritis of hip following fracture neck of femur and McMurray osteotomy. Note that the distal fragment is translated in relation to proximal fragment leading to off-ending of the canal in the two fragments. A spike of the proximal medial femoral cortex is occupying the metaphysis and will interfere with canal preparation. There is a posterior angulation in the lateral plane

Figures 5A and B: Check X-ray after THA using S-ROM stem and Pinnacle cup. Removal of intramedullary cortex and the use of modular stem allowed successful reconstruction without osteotomy

remaining femur or femoral component, or ideally, to both. The stability of the proximal segment is critically assessed with the broach or trial prosthesis in place. If questionable, internal fixation with a small plate is performed. A cortical strut graft medially and laterally may add stability to the construct.[15] An alternative could be to plan osteotomy with a step-cut configuration which gives inherent stability and

requires only circumferential wires or cables for additional support.

Hip resurfacing should be considered when there is a deformity of the proximal femur in the subtrochanteric region so that the insertion of a conventional stem would be impossible or require an osteotomy to realign the femur before an arthroplasty (Figures 6 A and B).

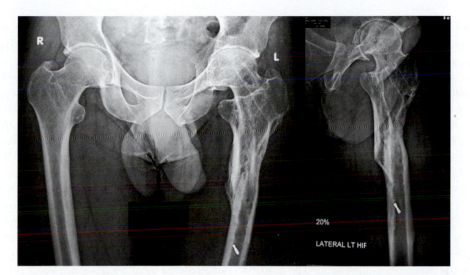

Figure 6A: Resurfacing should be considered in cases such as illustrated here, where there is marked proximal femoral deformity and resurfacing is not contraindicated

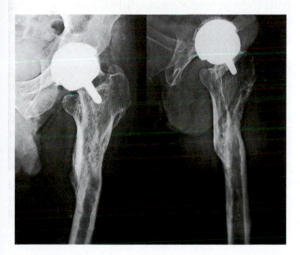

Figure 6B: Check X-ray after Birmingham hip resurfacing

Why an Spontaneous Rupture of Membranes Type of Modular Stem is Author's Implant of Choice in Cases of THA with Proximal Femoral Deformity?

Spontaneous rupture of membranes (S-ROM) modular stem prepares the proximal and distal portions of the femur independently, thus easily accommodating the issues of distorted proximal femoral anatomy, metaphyseal/diaphyseal mismatch, etc. S-ROM stem optimizes proximal and distal implant stability, allows maximal torsional stability during osteotomies (by virtue of the distal flutes).[4,5,16,17] This rotational stability allows rapid healing and weight bearing; therefore most surgeries can be performed in one stage.

S-ROM stem also permits easy adjustments to anteversion, offset and leg length to provide optimal biomechanical reconstruction of the deformed femur in THA. The S-ROM stem is available in standard +4, +6, +8 and +12 offset stems allowing establishment of optimum soft tissue tension without altering the limb length. Version can be easily adjusted too. Surgeon can place the proximal sleeve in a position maximizing contact with the proximal host bone and can place the stem in the position of optimum joint stability and optimal diaphyseal contact. S-ROM allows leg length equalization by adjustment offered at three levels—by adjusting the size and the depth of the insertion of the sleeve, by altering the length of the neck segment (calcar replacement necks are especially useful after osteotomy or when the sleeve has been inserted far too distally to achieve optimal bony contact), and, by altering the neck length using heads with different neck lengths. This versatility is especially useful in the face of severe proximal femoral deformities associated with significant leg length discrepancies.

In cases with developmental mismatch between metaphysis and diaphysis, modularity offered by S-ROM stem is ideal because 10 proximal sleeve sizes can be used with each femoral stem, allowing optimal proximal and distal fit and fill to occur independently. This feature allows its use even in Dorr C type of bone where large diameter stems and oversized sleeves maximize the proximal and distal contact and stability. The titanium stem with coronal slot reduces stem stiffness (and creation of stress riser at the tip of a stiff stem in an osteoporotic bone) associated with the large sizes. S-ROM hip stem creates less hoop stresses on potentially fragile stress risers from the screws and thin bone. The S-ROM stem also prepares a previously distorted anatomy by milling through the cortical bone that can occlude the femoral medullary canals and recreate proper femoral anteversion and reduces the risk of intraoperative or postoperative periprosthetic fracture due to the flexible titanium-slotted stem.

S-ROM prosthesis can be easily used with trochanteric fixation devices, including cable grips systems, wires or the S-ROM proximal trochanteric bolt.

Seung-Jae Lim et al[18] have reported a lower rate of complications with the use of S-ROM modular stem implant after joint-preserving procedures for osteonecrosis of the femoral head. In a cohort of 36 hips treated with S-ROM stem for failed joint-preserving procedures or osteonecrosis of femoral head, authors reported overall perioperative complication rate of 19% which is relatively low compared to 26% reported by Kawasaki et al[19] for THA following failed transtrochanteric rotational osteotomy. Authors felt that the S-ROM modular prosthesis in their series was able to accommodate the altered proximal femoral osteotomy caused by previous transtrochanteric osteotomy during the subsequent THA procedure.

RESULTS

The overall results reported for THA for proximal femoral deformities are worse than the THA done in patients where the proximal femur is not deformed. This is particularly true when the patient has had a varus producing intertrochanteric osteotomy.[8] The clinical results are worse when the medial displacement of the femoral shaft exceeds 10 mm. The valgus producing osteotomies usually produce minimal translation of the femoral shaft and most likely do not influence the surgery.[20,21] Ferguson and coworkers demonstrated failures in 15.8% of THA after a valgus intertrochanteric osteotomy at the end of 10 years follow-up compared to 29.9% failure rate after a varus osteotomy after an equal follow-up.[3]

Several authors have noticed higher failure rates with cemented stems post intertrochanteric osteotomy.[3,22,23] Cement mantle defects and use of small stems have been implicated in the diminished stem survival.[23] On the other hand, no failures were shown in 30 cases of THA with cementless stems done for post valgus intertrochanteric osteotomy for hip dysplasia at 7 years follow-up[21] and 4% failure rate in 48 hips at 16-year follow-up.[24]

High rates of failure have also been shown with the use of cemented stems along with subtrochanteric osteotomy with the results of second generation cementing techniques reported to be better than the first generation.[23] Using small stems to avoid reosteotomy of the deformity may not be the correct approach.[23] Osteotomy to correct the deformity is a better option for the surgeon.[3] The average time for the subtrochanteric osteotomy to heal completely has been reported to be 30 weeks[5,14,15,25] while nonunion of the reosteotomy sites has been reported in 13% cases.[5]

In conclusion, primary total hip arthroplasty is a common procedure that can present even the experienced surgeon with stiff challenge in the face of a proximal femoral deformity. Proper preoperative planning and availability of suitable implants are indispensable. Modular implants are extremely useful for most situations especially if a subtrochanteric osteotomy is required. Treatment must be individualized to address the level and the type of deformity, bone quality and the need for hardware removal. Moreover, surgeon experience and preference for the type of the implant to be used also should be taken into account.

REFERENCES

1. Benke GJ, Baker AS, Dounis E. Total hip replacement after upper femoral osteotomy. A clinical review. J Bone Joint Surg Br 1982;64:570-71.

2. Berry DJ. Total hip arthroplasty in patients with proximal femoral deformity. Clin Orthop 1999;369: 262-72.

3. Ferguson GM, Cabanela ME, Ilstrup DM. Total hip arthroplasty following failed intertrochanteric osteotomy. J Bone Joint Surg Br 1994;76B:252-7.

4. Ferdin H, Sanzin L, Sigurdsson B, Unander-Scharin L. Total hip arthroplasty in high congenital dislocation. 21 hips with a minimum five-year follow-up. J Bone Joint Surg Br 1991;73:430-2.

5. Papagelopoulos PJ, Trousdale RT, Lewallen DG. Total hip arthroplasty with femoral osteotomy for proximal femoral deformity. Clin Orthop 1996;332: 151-62.

6. Rittmeister M, Hanusek S, Starker M. Does tibial rotation correlate with femoral anteversion? Implications for hip arthroplasty. J Arthroplasty 2006;21:553-8.

7. Dupont JA, Baker AS, Dounis E. Low-friction arthroplasty of the hip for the failures of previous operations. J Bone Joint Surg Br 1972;54B:77-87.

8. Soballe K, Boll KL, Kofod S, Severinsen B, Kristensen SS. Total hip replacement after medial-displacement osteotomy of the proximal part of the femur. J Bone Joint Surg Am 1989;71A:692-7.

9. Barger W. Shape the implant to the patient: a rationale for the use of custom fit cementless total hip implants. Clin Orthop 1989;249:73-8.

10. Huo MH, Salvati ER, Lieberman JR, et al. Custom designed femoral prosthesis in total hip arthroplasty done with cement for severe dysplasia of the hip. J Bone Joint Surg 1993;75(A):1497-504.

11. Zhang B, Shiu KY, Wang M. Hip arthroplasty for failed internal fixation of intertrochanteric fractures. J Arthroplasty 2004;19:329-33.

12. Huo MH, Zatorski LE, Keggi KJ. Oblique femoral osteotomy in cementless total hip arthroplasty. Prospective consecutive series with a 3-year minimum follow-up period. J Arthroplasty 1995;10: 319-27.

13. Amstutz HC, Le Duff MJ. Hip resurfacing for other conditions and etiologies. Harlan C Amstutz (Ed). In Hip Resurfacing, Principles, Indications, Techniques and Results. Philadelphia:Saunders, Elsevier. 2008; pp. 227-8.

14. Zadeh HG, Hua J, Walker PS, Muirhead-Allwood SK. Uncemented total hip arthroplasty with subtrochanteric derotational osteotomy for severe femoral anteversion. J Arthroplasty 1999;14:686.

15. Glassman AH, Engh CA, Bobyn JD. Proximal femoral osteotomy as an adjunct in cementless revision total hip arthroplasty. J Arthroplasty 1987; 2:47-63.

16. Bruce WJ, Rizkallah SM, Kwon YM, Goldberg JA, Walsh WR. A new technique of subtrochanteric shortening in total hip arthroplasty: surgical technique and results of 9 cases. J Arthroplasty 2000; 15:617-26.

17. Chareancholvanich K, Becker DA, Gustilo RP. Treatment of congenital dislocated hip by arthroplasty with femoral shortening. Clin Orthop 1999;360:127-35.

18. Seung-Jae Lim, Young-Wan Moon, Sang-Soo Eun, Youn-Soo Park. Total hip arthroplasty using the S-ROM modular stem after joint-preserving procedures for osteonecrosis of the femoral head. J Arthroplasty 2008;23(4):495-501.

19. Kawasaki M, Hasegawa Y, Sakano S, et al. Total hip arthroplasty after failed transtrochanteric rotational osteotomy for avascular necrosis of the femoral head. J Arthroplasty 2005;20:574.

20. Iwase T, Hasegawa Y, Iwasada S, et al. Total hip arthroplasty after failed intertrochanteric valgus osteotomy for advanced osteoarthrosis. Clin Orthop 1999;364:175-81.

21. Suzuki K, Kawachi S, Matsubara M, et al. Cementless total hip replacement after previous intertrochanteric valgus osteotomy for advanced osteoarthritis. J Bone Joint Surg Br 2007;89:1155-7.

22. Boos N, Krushell R, Ganz R, et al. Total hip arthroplasty after previous proximal femoral osteotomy. J Bone Joint Surg Br 1997:247-53.

23. Shinar AA, Harris WH. Cemented total hip arthroplasty following previous femoral osteotomy: an average 16-year follow-up study. J Arthroplasty 1998;13:243-53.

24. Parsch D, Jung AW, Thomsen M, et al. Good survival of uncemented tapered stems for failed intertrochanteric osteotomy: a mean 16 year follow-up study in 45 patients. Arch Orthop Trauma Surg 2008;128(10):1081-5.

25. Park MS, Kin KH, Jeong WC. Transverse subtrochanteric shortening osteotomy in primary total hip arthroplasty for patients with severe hip developmental dysplasia. J Arthroplasty 2007; 22:1031-6.

15 | Computer-assisted Navigation in Complex Primary Total Hip Arthroplasty

Kamal Deep

INTRODUCTION

Computer-assisted navigation has been one of the most important developments in the recent times in orthopedics. While the joint replacement arthroplasty became popular and developed through 1960s to 1990s, the most striking change in 21st century seems to be better understanding of the kinematics and dynamics of the joints. Use of computer-assisted surgery has played a vital role in this field and taken us a step further in putting the theoretical preoperative plan into practical operative action giving feedback real-time to the surgeon.

Historically the use in orthopedics started from spinal surgery, building on from neurosurgical navigation. The use of computer assistance in joint arthroplasty came about in early 1990s when robotic joint replacements were attempted. Then followed the use of computer-assisted navigation. Although both use computers, there is a peculiar difference in robotic surgery and computer navigation as the former is performed by mainly robots and the latter mainly by surgeons. Nowadays, there are attempts to combine the two and exploit the advantages of both.

The main process of computer navigation involves registration of the individual anatomy to the computer, attachment of rigid bodies (trackers) to the bones and instruments and real time tracking of these rigid bodies in space via infrared waves or electromagnetic media or other means.

Use of computer-assisted surgery (CAS) in total hip replacement (THR) is recent and is gaining more popularity though a bit less than in total knee arthroplasty. The main reason for this is that a lot of misplaced implants do not cause as many immediate

visible problems as they can cause in the TKR. But as time goes by surgeons are realizing its potential advantages in the THR by getting good results. The problems with conventional techniques in THR surgery that are related to implant malposition and include dislocation, impingement, leg length discrepancy and early failure[1-3] Impingement has been highlighted recently to be a big problem especially with use of ceramics.[3,4] Also with metal-on metal bearings the metal ion concentration is much more with malplaced implants.[5] Malposition of the acetabulum in hip resurfacing arthroplasty can lead to disastrous consequences of adverse reaction to metal debris like ALVAL reaction and pseudo-tumors, which has led to a visible decline in the frequency of the resurfacing metal hip replacements.[6] There is no consensus on the standard position where the acetabular cup should be placed, although some safe zones like Lewinnek have been described.[7] The functional plane may be different for every individual and there can be contractures of various degrees in the arthritic hip leading to different degrees of pelvic tilt. This also holds true for conventional surgery.

Most of the computer navigation systems presently use anterior pelvic plane as the reference plane for registering the anatomy of the pelvis. This is acquired by registering the two anterior superior iliac spines (ASIS) and pubic symphysis. While this plane gives consistent fixed bony points, it may not represent a true reference for every individual functional position due to the variation in pelvic tilt. Alternatives have been explored but have not been proved to be better than anterior pelvic plane. These include posterior superior iliac spines and transverse acetabular ligament. Recently inherent acetabular axis has been taken as a reference to denote the anatomy of the acetabulum.[8] This is defined by three points taken on the acetabular margin; the superior point is taken on a line joining the iliac tubercle with acetabular notch, anterior and posterior points at the widest profile of the acetabulum. The author claims it to give consistently good results.[8] Most common difficulty with anterior pelvic plane is registration in imageless navigation, especially if the surgeon uses lateral position for the surgery. While THR in primary osteoarthritis is relatively better understood and gives good results using conventional techniques, the complexity increases if the arthritis is secondary to an underlying cause. In complex primary THR, the anatomy of the hip is distorted leading to loss of the available usual landmarks. In this situation, it is highly desirable that the surgeon gets maximum guidance from any sources available. CAS can play a vital role in these hips. Not only can it guide the surgeon on orientation of the components but also the positioning of the center of the hip, are visible at the time of operation, where the surgeon can make important decisions in the placement of components. These are very important in dysplastic hips and the hips destroyed by trauma, infection, inflammation and malignancy.

Potential Advantages

Computer-assisted surgery (CAS) gives surgeon individual patient specific anatomy based on which one can formulate the plan to make the bone preparation and produce optimum result. For the acetabular cup it can show real time in what orientation the surgeon is placing the cup in 6 degrees of freedom. It can give inclination, anteversion, flexion, any anteroposterior, mediolateral and superoinferior shifts that the surgeon produces and can correct them at the time of surgery. Similarly for the femoral stem it can show the flexion/extension, varus/valgus, anteversion/retroversion, offset and leg length change. Most of the systems available should be able to show above parameters but some may differ. The surgeon is advised to look at these in detail before making a choice of the system he/she would like to use.

It has been proved in various studies that it increases the accuracy of anatomical placement as compared to conventional means even in experienced hands.[1] It has also been shown to correct leg length discrepancy better than conventional techniques.[3,9] Thus, problems with conventional surgery that are related to implant malposition should be addressed by this.

The pelvis can move during the procedure without knowledge or control of the surgeon under the drapes leading to chances of misplacement of the cup. With navigation, any movement of the pelvis will be detected by the computer and the chances of misplacement are minimal.

It is thus hoped that it can prevent early failures and potentially lead to better function and increased survival of the implants. As the CAS techniques are in infancy it is too early to state if this will hold true, but it does appeal to common sense based on the early findings in the literature.

It has been shown to be helpful in training young surgeons and can give consistent results in trainees' hands which compare well with experienced surgeons.[10] It is also helpful if minimally invasive approaches are being used where the field of view is limited.[11]

It guides the surgeon through various stages of the procedure and shows real time what he/she is doing.

Operative Technique

We describe here the technique used in imageless registration method which is most commonly used technique. Only the steps which are important from navigation point of view are described. One must know how to do a conventional hip replacement arthroplasty. It involves various stages as in conventional surgery. The method described here is one we use but there can be variations with different surgeons and commercial systems available. At present there are not many dedicated softwares available for complex or revision hips, so in most situations primary total hip software is used and seems to serve the purpose though in revisions, we do need dedicated instrumentation directed to the procedure. There is dedicated software available for dysplastic hips from Orthopilot (B Braun Aesculap, Tuttlingen, Germany).

Preoperative Planning

Preoperative planning is essential, especially in complex primary THR. One has to determine before the start of the operation, based on radiological and clinical criteria, in what direction and to what extent a change in the center of the hip is desired and what change in offset and leg length does the patient need. It is also important to note the anatomy of the acetabulum, if needed by supplementing with a preoperative CT scan, the position, thickness and any deficiency of the walls of the acetabular cavity. The femoral version, shape and medullary canal dimensions should also be considered.

System Set-up

Patient and part preparation is done as in conventional surgery. Position of the patient can be supine or lateral. The limb is prepared from lower chest to foot and left in clear view. It is important that one can access the knee, iliac crest and pelvis for proper registration of anatomy and attaching the trackers to the bone. In obese individuals if one is using the lateral position with posterior approach, it may be easier to leave the patient first in sloppy lateral position till registration of the pelvis is done and then tighten the posterior supports. Echocardiographic patches with central knobs may also be used to guide the contralateral ASIS and pubic symphysis under the drapes for registration of the pelvic plane.

Patient data and side are fed into the system. The trackers and instruments are registered and calibrated if needed by the system. The trackers are attached to pelvis and femur with various means depending on the system being used (Figure 1). The site of attachment for pelvis can be iliac crest or supra-acetabular area. The femoral tracker may be attached either to the trochanteric region or distally shaft away from the main operative incision. The means of attachment vary from 1 to 3 pins to a square nail. Whatever means is used, it should be a secure and stable fixation not interfering with main operation itself. The camera (Figure 2) is adjusted so that it can look at both the trackers and is at a proper distance (usually varies between 1.6 and 2.5 meters from surgical field) to be out of surgical field and give accurate readings. Normally the computer

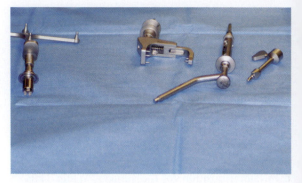

Figure 1: The tracker attachment devices for the pelvic (supra-acetabular area) and femoral (C-clamp for trochanteric region) rigid bodies

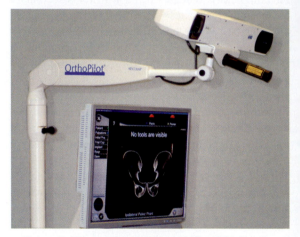

Figure 2: The camera is adjusted in the right direction and distance from the operative site

screen will indicate if the camera cannot see any of the trackers properly.

Registration of Pelvis and Acetabulum

This can be image based or imageless. In the image-based method preoperative CT scan or fluoroscopy may be used. We use imageless method of registration. The pelvis is registered by frontal plane constituted by the two anterior superior iliac spines and pubic tubercles or pubic symphysis. These points are intact in most of the complex primary hips; hence act as a good reference for orientation. Some systems also register a functional plane constituted by midaxillary point and greater trochanter in neutral position of the leg. This can be difficult to reproduce as both these points are not single discrete bony points and thus are open to errors. The hip joint is then exposed as in conventional surgery, neck osteotomy performed and head part extracted. The acetabular registration is done by denoting the true medial wall (Floor), acetabular surface and/or circumference of the margin. This will give an approximate diameter of the acetabulum and a native anatomy. A cup trial or reamer of the same diameter as the acetabulum can be used to insert in the acetabulum and the center of the reamer is thus registered by computer as the center of hip. The orientation of the inherent acetabulum can also be thus recorded. This center acts as a reference for further calculations. It is important to note that in complex hips the acetabular anatomy is not that clear and the preoperative planning comes into play. The local acetabular anatomy may not be much help for orienting the acetabular cup in complex hips.

Femoral Registration

There are different methods used by different systems. The anterior midpatellar point and anterior midpoint of the ankle with a knee bent to 90° is used by one system. With another system trochanteric fossa is registered first followed by popliteal fossa which can be registered either as a single point or by registering two femoral epicondyles. Then the knee is bent to ninety degrees to avoid any effect of leg rotation and midpoint of the Achilles tendon is registered. This forms a virtual femoral plane by combining all these points to act as a reference for the femoral components. One has to consider the inherent anatomy of the femur and be vigilant these are the planes generated by computer to give orientation between different registered points. It ignores the intervening shaft anatomy which may be bent especially if there are any previous fractures or malformations. The surgeon needs to take that in consideration.

Acetabular Cup

Acetabular reamers are then used to prepare the cup bed after good exposure is achieved. The reamer handle is attached with a tracker (Figure 3) which communicates with the computer to give orientation and position of the reamer in all 6 degrees of freedom including inclination, version, flexion, superoinferior, anteroposterior and mediolateral position (Figure 4). Reaming is executed in accordance with the preoperative plan. Similar information is given when the cup is inserted as a tracker is attached to the cup insertion handle. For the uncemented cups it is important to be very careful when preparing with the reamers to be in correct orientation. For the cemented cups one can change the position of the cup within the cement mantle to some extent before it sets.

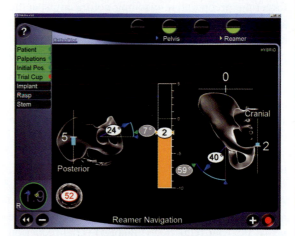

Figure 3: The active tracker is attached to the pelvis and passive tracker with reflective balls is attached to the reamer handle for acetabular reaming

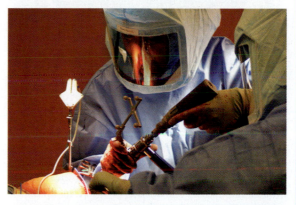

Figure 4: The acetabular reaming screen showing the reamer size, anteroposterior, mediolateral and craniocaudal position. It also shows the inclination, anteversion and distance to the true floor

COMPUTER-ASSISTED NAVIGATION IN COMPLEX PRIMARY TOTAL HIP ARTHROPLASTY

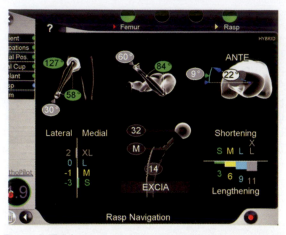

Figure 5: The femoral rasping showing internal and external rotations that will be achieved by the shown anteversion of the rasp position. The lower part of the screen shows virtual trial including the offset, size of the head, neck and stem and the change it will make to the leg length

Femoral Stem

The femur is prepared in conventional fashion taking care of the correct orientation which is shown by the computer as the tracker is attached to the femoral broach handle. It shows the position in all 6° of freedom including flexion, varus, version, offset and lengthening (Figure 5). Similar readings are given when inserting stem component. It is important not to forget the preoperative planning noting any specific anomalies in the femoral shape. In some softwares it can even give the virtual range of motion a specific position of the femoral component will produce and thus can help plan the version of the component. Again in uncemented stems it is important to be careful at the time of preparation of bed. In cemented stems one can alter the position to some extent in the cement mantle.

Final Steps

A virtual reduction can be done and effect of various lengths of femoral neck can be seen even without the actual hip trial reduction (Figure 5). Trial reduction is then done with selected component and the new hip center seen. A change of leg length and offset can be seen which can be changed to an extent even

at this stage by varying the neck length. The final range of movements and points of impingement are recorded in the computer and procedure finished as in conventional technique.

A lot of development in the CAS technology specific to THR also needs to take place before it is accepted as a conventional technique by all. The present methods need to be modified; the instrumentation needs to be directed to CAS and a whole new range of implants need to be made to properly reproduce the optimal biomechanics. The registration process needs to be simplified and the reference plane needs to be standardized also taking into the account the pelvic tilt in various postures.

Issues

While the accuracy of the computer navigation systems in laboratory environment is up to last degree and millimeter, this precision does not always translate into the operating environment. There are issues which need attention.

REGISTRATION

Registration of patient anatomy is the main issue affecting the accuracy of navigated surgery. In image-based techniques of registration it may not be as much of a problem, but these use more manpower, radiation and are more expensive. In imageless techniques the accuracy of registration may be questionable.[12] It can be difficult to acquire anterior pelvic plane using ASIS and pubic symphysis, especially in obese patients when the surgeon operates in lateral position. Therefore, surgeons are searching for reference points and planes other than the anterior pelvic plane. The effects of wrong registration are shown in Table 1 (craniocaudal direction), and Table 2 (transverse plane anteroposterior direction). A wrong registration in mediolateral direction of the ASIS does not affect the inclination or version of the cup. As can be seen an error of up to 2 cm of anterior superior iliac spine (ASIS) registration in most cases affect the orientation to only up to 1° to 4°. The one most important point affecting the accuracy is the accuracy of registration in transverse plane (depth)

Table 1: Showing the change in inclination and anteversion of the acetabular cup of an average pelvis (with distance between ASIS being 240 mm) with right side being the treatment side effects of wrong registration in craniocaudal direction

- Right ASIS – Cranial (+)/Caudal (–) Shift (mm)	Actual cup position	
	Inclination (°)	Anteversion (°)
30	52	18
25	51	18
20	49	19
15	48	19
10	47	19
5	46	20
0	45	20
– 5	44	20
– 10	43	21
– 15	42	21
– 20	41	22
– 25	39	22
– 30	38	22

- Left ASIS – Cranial (+)/Caudal (–) Shift (mm)	Actual cup position	
	Inclination (°)	Anteversion (°)
30	38	22
25	39	22
20	41	22
15	42	21
10	43	21
5	44	20
0	45	20
– 5	46	20
– 10	47	19
– 15	48	19
– 20	49	19
– 25	51	18
– 30	52	18

Table 2: The change in inclination and anteversion of the acetabular cup of an average pelvis (with distance between ASIS being 240 mm) with right side being the treatment side effects of wrong registration in transverse plane

- Right ASIS – Anterior (+)/Posterior (–) Shift (mm)	Actual cup position	
	Inclination (°)	Anteversion (°)
30	43	18
25	43	18
20	43	19
15	44	19
10	44	19
5	44	20
0	45	20
– 5	46	20
– 10	46	21
– 15	47	21
– 20	47	21
– 25	48	21
– 30	49	21

- Left ASIS – Anterior (+)/Posterior (–) Shift (mm)	Actual cup position	
	Inclination (°)	Anteversion (°)
30	43	3
25	43	6
20	43	9
15	44	12
10	44	15
5	44	17
0	45	20
– 5	46	23
– 10	46	25
– 15	47	28
– 20	47	30
– 25	48	33
– 30	49	35

for the contralateral ASIS as this can affect the anteversion to a huge extent.

TRACKER-RELATED PROBLEMS

There is a potential for tracker attachment site morbidity as one has to make a hole in the bone to attach the trackers to the bone. This may potentially lead to fracture, though none has been reported in the literature yet associated with THR navigation.

If one is using the passive tracker, the contamination with fluid or blood can affect the visibility and computer may not recognize the tracker.

If the tracker attaching pins are not positioned carefully, there can be neurovascular damage, though none has been reported yet.

The trackers have a potential to move as the pelvis can be porotic in old patients in whom generally the THR is performed. If using single pins there can be rotary movement. In an experiment carried out at the University of Brisbane,[13] the authors found larger diameter pins had a better hold though 4 and 5 mm ratchet pins did not show much difference (150-200 N). Double cortical pins had a better hold as compared to single cortical pins. Triple pin fixation of a tripod, bone to pin fixation did not fail before failure of the metal of tripod itself. Pullout strength was much stronger (10-15 times) than the translational strength. A registrar/assistant can produce forces measured up to 150 Newtons with sudden bump as well as sustained force which was much less than the forces required to pull out the tracker pin, just less than translating a 4 or 5 mm diameter pin but more than the required forces to rotate the tracker.[13] Thus, choice of the tracker attaching device is important.

TIME

The procedure may take longer than conventional technique. In the beginning it can be up to 30 minutes longer. This comes down to about 10 minutes after doing up to fifty cases, once the learning curve is over. The operating environment, experience and familiarity of the operating staff also have a bearing on the speed of the operation. Author operating time of a typical primary navigated THR is 50 to 60 minutes.

OUTCOME MEASURES

Mostly the postoperative outcome of the components is evaluated with plain radiographs in routine practice. These are not as accurate as the CT scan or computer navigation itself. It is important to have outcome measures for evaluation, which can simulate the sensitivity of computer navigation.

FUTURE OF COMPUTER-ASSISTED SURGERY

It is opinion of the author that the technology will be much simpler and user-friendly in future. Software and instrumentations are being designed to cater for complex situations and revision procedures at the time of writing this chapter. It will be used for all the joint arthroplasties and most of other orthopedic surgeries including deformity correction, spinal, trauma and tumor surgery. It will be used even for preoperative and postoperative evaluation of kinematics, implants and track their progress with time recognizing early failures before it happens. It is also going to be helpful in training surgeons and can act as an evaluating tool for examination purposes. Its potential for research and understanding of biomechanics of humans is huge and will no doubt assist us give better outcomes for our patients.

REFERENCES

1. Wixson RL. Computer-assisted total hip navigation. Instr Course Lect. 2008;57:707-20.
2. Ecker TM, Murphy SB. Application of surgical navigation to total hip arthroplasty. Proc Inst Mech Eng [H]. 2007;221(7):699-712.
3. Sugano N, Nishii T, Miki H, Yoshikawa H, Sato Y, Tamura S. Mid-term results of cementless total hip replacement using a ceramic-on-ceramic bearing with and without computer navigation. J Bone Joint Surg Br. 2007;89(4):455-60.
4. Murali R, Bonar SF, Kirsh G, Walter WK, Walter WL. Osteolysis in third-generation alumina ceramic-on-ceramic hip bearings with severe impingement and titanium metallosis. J Arthroplasty 2008;23(8):1240. e13-9. Epub 2008.
5. Onda K, Nagoya S, Kaya M, Yamashita T. Cup-neck impingement due to the malposition of the implant as a possible mechanism for metallosis in

metal-on-metal total hip arthroplasty. Orthopaedics. 2008;31(4):396.

6. Langton DJ, Joyce TJ, Jameson SS, et al. Adverse reaction to metal debris following hip resurfacing– The influence of component type, orientation and volumetric wear. J Bone Joint Surg Br. 2011; 93B(2):164-71.

7. Lewinnek GE, Lewis JL, Tarr R, Compere CL, Zimmerman JR. Dislocations after total hip-replacement arthroplasties. J Bone Joint Surg Am. 1978;60(2):217-20.

8. Hakki S, Bilotta V, Oliveira D, Dordelly L. Acetabular central axis: is it the future of hip navigation? Orthopaedics. 2010;33(10 Suppl):43-7.

9. Confalonieri N, Manzotti A, Montironi F, Pullen C. Leg length discrepancy, dislocation rate, and offset in total hip replacement using a short modular stem: navigation vs conventional freehand. Orthopaedics. 2008;31(10 Suppl 1).

10. Gofton W, Dubrowski A, Tabloie F, Backstein D. The effect of computer navigation on trainee learning of surgical skills. J Bone Joint Surg Am. 2007;89(12):2819-27.

11. Judet H. Five years of experience in hip navigation using a mini-invasive anterior approach. Orthopaedics. 2007;30(10 Suppl):S141-3.

12. Pinoit Y, May O, Girard J, Laffargue P, Ala Eddine T, Migaud H. Low accuracy of anterior pelvic plane to guide the position of the cup with imageless computer assistance. Variation of position in 106 patients. Rev Chir Orthop Reparatrice Appar Mot. 2007;93(5):455-60.

13. Deep K, Ward N, Donnelly W, Tevelan G, Crawford R. Biomechanical force displacement analysis of strength of fixation of tracker holding devices to bone in computer aided joint replacements. J Bone Joint Surg Br. 2006 Sep;88B(Supp):439.

COMPUTER-ASSISTED NAVIGATION IN COMPLEX PRIMARY TOTAL HIP ARTHROPLASTY

16 | Evaluation of Patients with Pain after Total Hip Arthroplasty

Mandeep S Dhillon, Sarvdeep S Dhatt

Total hip replacement (THR) is fast becoming one of the most commonly performed orthopedic surgeries in modern times. According to the US National Center for Health statistics annually, more than 168,000 primary and 30,000 revision total hip replacements are performed in the United States;[1] the trend is increasing in Asian countries also, but specific statistics are not available. With the advent of newer technologies and advances we have come to the stage when even the most debilitating conditions can be fairly treated by arthroplasty. According to the American Association of Hip and Knee surgeons there may be a need for 500,000 hip replacements and 3,000,000 knee replacements each year by the year 2030. With people living longer than ever, arthritis of the hip and knee is more common and the number of cyclic loads per hip may be touch around 10 million per year;[2-4] this longevity means that the implant may have to last longer, without any clinical symptoms.

Once a hip is implanted, the good outcomes depend upon many factors ranging from good gait, deformity correction, leg length and most importantly cessation of pain. Incomplete satisfaction often stems from pain around the surgical site or deep inside the joint leading to significant debate regarding the assessment of a good outcome in hip arthroplasty. Britton et al.[5] recommended using the presence or absence of pain as an indicator of the success of total hip replacement. Many hip questionnaires have been developed for this purpose; the Harris Hip Score[6] (which was developed in 1969) assesses pain, function, range of motion, and absence of deformity, and is the leading evaluation tool. Others include the Oxford Hip Score[7] which is a 12-item questionnaire for patients undergoing THR. It was developed from patient interviews and validated against the SF-36 and the Health Assessment Questionnaire.

According to an instructional lecture[8] of the American Academy of Orthopedic Surgeons (AAOS), pain following total hip replacement is difficult to assess because it is subjective and is often underweighted on commonly used hip scoring systems. They recommended that the pain and function of the hip scale, developed on the basis of the recommendation of the Société Internationale de Chirurgie Orthopédique et de Traumatologie (SICOT), represents an attempt to overcome these limitations by more careful weighting and measurement of pain.[9, 10]

EVALUATION OF THE PATIENT

It is very important to have a systematic approach to a patient with the complaint of pain following a hip arthroplasty. This should include a very detailed history of the patient's preoperative complaints to the presenting complaints following the arthroplasty, physical examination of the patient. There should be a comprehensive investigation of the patient which should include the laboratory blood check-up, radiology and interventional tests such as arthrography and aspiration cytology. These tests will be discussed in detail as we go along.

Patient Evaluation

One of the important issues to consider in evaluating the patient is the type of implant used. Postoperative issues may be different in bipolar or monopolar arthroplasty, as well in cemented and uncemented implants. Pain after revision is a different issue altogether. For the present chapter, the authors will focus on primary total hip arthroplasty, both cemented and uncemented types, leaving out the bipolar and the revision options. Other considerations would include timing of the pain (early or late postoperative), pre-existing comorbidities, pain type as well as actual localization of the pain.

History and Differential Diagnosis

Groin pain is the commonest presentation after THA. The differential diagnosis of groin pain in this scenario includes septic and aseptic loosening of the acetabular component,[11,12] occult pubic ramus fracture,[13,14] neurologic,[15,16] vascular lesions,[17] heterotopic ossification[18] and referred pain from the spine,[19,20] knee, retroperitoneum, or abdomen. Tendinopathies [21] also have been identified as a cause of pain after THR.

Many a times we have seen that there may be a coexisting disease other than the hip pathology, such as a spine issue, which may have been overlooked at the time of surgery. It is quite common in cases of degenerative elderly patients to have some sort of superadded degenerative spine problem such as canal stenosis.[19] These cases may not see a cessation of pain after the surgery; a patient with postoperative pain need a detailed work up, including a detailed neurological examination, to delineate the exact source of pain. A comprehensive history also helps us to determine the exact source and site of pain; the exact localization of pain site is an indirect indicator of the underlying pathology. This may vary from trochanteric bursitis secondary to the underlying sutures or hardware, or pain over the buttocks indicating some sort of facetal hypertrophy, etc. Trochanteric bursitis, or lateral trochanteric pain, is a known complication of total hip arthroplasty, with reported rates ranging from 4-17%.[22-25] Distally occurring pain over the thigh is usually related to femoral stem loosening.[26]

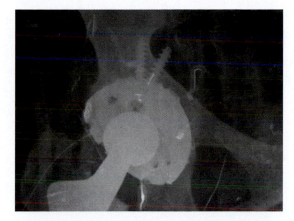

Figure 1: Long screw causing causalgic pain

Early pain in the immediate postoperative period may be neurological in origin. With screw fixation of acetabular cups becoming common place, irritation of the sciatic nerve due to long screws (Figure 1) may lead to neuralgic pain along the areas of distribution of the nerve. Stretch pain may occur in the femoral distribution when excessive flexion deformity is corrected at surgery, or in sciatic distribution if leg length correction exceeds 3 cm or so.

Any history of persistent discharge or wound problems after surgery may indicate an underlying infection. Pain on rest and at night raises suspicion of infection; persistent low-level pain following a hip replacement is consistent with an occult infection.[27] If there has been a pain free interval after the surgery then causes such as loosening, infection and implant failure should be kept in mind. After ruling out localized causes it is very important to correlate the pain with any systemic manifestation such as weight loss, low grade fever, anorexia or malaise which may again indicate other underlying chronic conditions. Rare causes of pain should also be kept in mind; we have seen late onset pain in well fixed implants occurring due to bone metastases around the stem (Figure 2).

The causes of postoperative pain may be divided into early and late depending upon the site (Table 1).

PHYSICAL EXAMINATION

The physical examination of the patient should be done after a detailed history, which allows focus on

Table 1: Causes of postoperative pain

Early	Late
Infection	Loosening
Intraoperative fracture	Thigh pain
Muscular tendonitis	Stress fracture
Irritation of psoas	Pubic rami, sacral fractures
Stretching of adductors	Nonunion of trochanteric osteotomy
Vastus lateralis herniation	Heterotopic ossification
Trochanteric bursitis/tear gluteus medius	Lumbar/knee/pelvic/abdominal pathology
Nerve injury	Prosthesis failure
	Instability

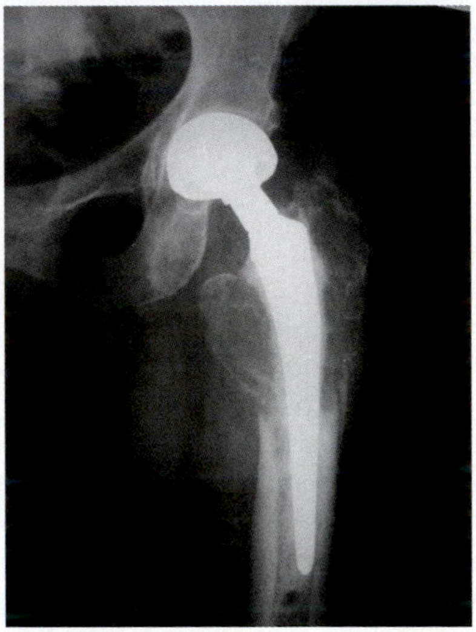

Figure 2: Pain due to bony metastases around the implant

a specific issue and having some sort of differential diagnosis in hand. Pain associated with movement may indicate loosening, especially when it occurs in extremes of motion range. In infection and implant failure there will be pain throughout the motion range. Thus, the relevance and importance of a detailed physical examination cannot be understated.

Patient evaluation starts from the most important aspect of observation, which includes the gait pattern. The gait should be observed so that full stride length can be observed from the frontal and sagittal planes. Common keypoints to be focused on include the stride length, stance phase, foot rotation (internal/external progression angle), pelvic rotation in the x and y axes, Trendelenburg gait, antalgic gait patterns, leg length issues and pelvic wink. The pelvic wink demonstrates excessive rotation in axial plane greater than the normal 40° toward the affected hip to obtain terminal hip extension. This gait pattern is associated with internal hip pathology and secondary hip flexion contracture. Patient usually point to specific areas where pain occurs during walking.

Shoulder heights should then be observed, along with the iliac crest levels, to further address leg length issues. It is routine to measure the distance from the anterior-superior iliac spine to medial malleolus and record any length discrepancy. Forward bending allows the inspection of the spine from behind and identifies scoliosis, and lateral inspection of the lumbar spine reveals any excessive lordosis or paravertebral muscle spasm. A tight iliopsoas will produce an increase in the lumbar lordosis, similar to the finding in neuromuscular disease.

Trendelenburg's test should be performed on both legs, first nonaffected and then the diseased one, to help establish a baseline neuro-proprioceptive function. The Trendelenburg's test is helpful in testing not only the strength of the abductor mechanism, but also the entire affective/effective loop. It is good if preoperative data about this test is available to act as a reference point.

Pain due to neural issues is rare; the pattern is typical and findings are specific. Neurologic evaluation is also very important as there are chances of nerve injuries in hip arthroplasty which occur about less than one percent of all primary total hip arthroplasty.[28] The nerve injury may occur due to the retractors or screws, and even limb length inequality. The motor assessment of the obturator, superior gluteal, sciatic and femoral nerve function is graded on a standard 0 to 4/4 scale. Sensations of the L2 through S1 segments should be tested and should be compared with the contralateral limb.

The straight leg raise should be performed to aid in the diagnosis of radicular etiologies. The deep tendon reflexes are recorded in traditional fashion at the Achilles and patellar region and graded 0 to 4/4. The pulses of the dorsalis pedis and posterior tibialis are recorded as present or absent. The skin and lymphatics are inspected, compared, and any scarring of extremity noted. The surgical site is noted for any induration, erythema and drainage. The internal and external rotation measurements of the hip are recorded in the sitting position to have a stable and fixed angle of 90° at the hip joint. Osseous constraint pathology, such as femoroacetabular impingement, or rotational constraint from increased or decreased femoral acetabular anteversion, can result in significant differences between sides. Increase in femoral or acetablular anteversion usually demonstrates an increase in the internal rotation.

Hip instability due to wear or loosening is an important cause of pain when seen late. In our country, many people delay follow-up after a settled prosthesis and may present with frank loosening (Figure 3) or a dislocating prosthesis (Figure 4), which has been symptomatic for long periods of time.

This battery of clinical tests helps to begin further distinction of internal versus extra-articular sources of dysfunction. The Thomas test is used to demonstrate the presence of a hip flexion contracture. Patrick (FABER) is the classic examination for the distinction of hip pain with rotation in the abducted position, opposing the anterior-superior rim of the femoral neck adjacent to the 12-o'clock position of the acetabulum. Pain may be referred to the spine or the sacroiliac joint directing further evaluation to these areas.

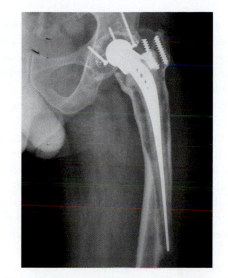

Figure 3: Aseptic loosening around the implant

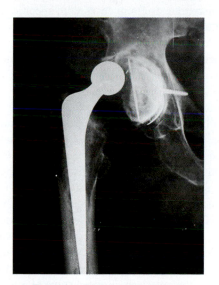

Figure 4: Dislocated prosthesis

The abdominal examination should include the basics of inspection, palpation for mass or fascial hernia, which can be assessed by isometric contraction of the rectus abdominis and obliques. The ilioinguinal region should be inspected; Tinel's at the femoral nerve and palpation of the femoral pulse are assessed. Palpation for abdominal or iliofemoral mass should be performed on all patients. Palpation of the adductor tubercle as the patient adducts the extended leg may help identify adductor tendonitis.

Palpation of the sacroiliac joint, gluteus maximus origin, piriformis, sciatic nerve, iliotibial band, greater trochanteric bursae, tensor fascia lata, and ischial tuberosity are performed to locate the exact area of discomfort. The Ober's test, flexion adduction internal rotation test, and the abduction extension external rotation complete the five tests in the lateral position. The Ober's test is performed in both the extended hip with the knee flexed in traditional fashion, as well as with the shoulders rotated back toward the table starting with the knee straight to assess the gluteus maximus contribution to the iliotibial band. Knee flexion may decrease the pain at the maximus origin in cases with specific gluteus maximus contracture. The gluteus medius tone can be graded with the iliotibial band and released with the knee in flexion, which aids in the diagnosis of medius tears. Patients with large tears will not be able to raise the leg even against gravity.

Scour's test can also be performed in the supine position; this attempts to elicit pain or clicking with passive flexion through an arc of external rotation to internal rotation. The abduction extension external rotation test is comparable to the apprehension test in the shoulder. The knee is straight with the hip abducted at 30°, in neutral rotation, and brought from 10° flexion to terminal extension externally rotating the straight leg while pushing forward on the greater trochanter to reproduce any complaint of pain or discomfort. A positive test is relief of the pain once the anteriorly directed force is released. A positive test can be associated with microinstability or combined anterior anteversion, acetabular anteversion summation.

LABORATORY INVESTIGATIONS

The various blood tests which should be carried out include:
• Complete hemogram
• Total leukocyte counts

• Differential leukocyte counts. The leukocyte count is of little use for diagnosing infection at the site of a total hip replacement.[29]

ESR: Erythrocyte sedimentation rate (ESR) useful in the diagnosis of infection when there is no other reason for ESR elevation. It is usually elevated in septic THR cases. In greater than 85% of patients with infection after THR have elevation of ESR and 79% have a rate of more than 50 mm/hour; however surgery itself causes some elevation and a preoperative baseline value is of help during the early postoperative phase when infection is suspected. In late developing pain, ESR is usually significant, especially in nonrheumatoid hips with generalized inflammatory pathologies.

Screening levels: If 30 to 35 mm is used as a threshold for infection, then the sensitivity rate will range from 61 to 88% and the specificity rate will range from 96 to 100%.

Normal values: ESR rate in patients undergoing an uncomplicated THR reaches maximum of 64 mm/hour on 6 postoperative days; rates averaged 50 mm/hour until 3 weeks after surgery and thereafter slowly decreased to 30 mm/hour over course of year; after 3 weeks, rate that remains higher than 40 mm/hour suggests that patient has infection until proved otherwise; polymethylmethacrylate does not appear to have significant effect on ESR, and increase that occurs after uncomplicated THR is related to surgical intervention.

C-reactive protein: (may be more sensitive than ESR–10 mg per liter is used as the threshold for infection). It has been seen that that levels consistently returned to normal within three weeks after a successful hip replacement.[30] The measurement of both the ESR and the C-reactive protein (CRP) level had only one false-negative result in a series of twenty-three patients with an infection.[31] The combined efficacy of these two measurements was also confirmed in a study which showed that a normal CRP level and a normal ESR were 100% specific for excluding infection.[32]

In our institute, it is a protocol to have a baseline quantitative CRP done in all cases preoperatively. This helps in those cases of THR in which the

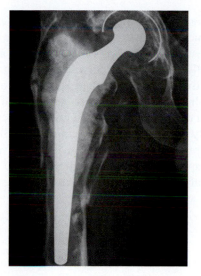

Figure 5: Loosening of the prosthesis

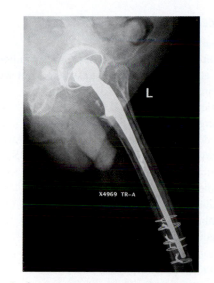

Figure 6: Septic loosening show radiolucent lines around the prosthesis and endosteal scalloping around the collar

preoperative diagnosis is rheumatoid arthritis where we would expect a high baseline CRP. Sustained high levels, with persistence of pain and associated fever, assume significance.

ROLE OF RADIOLOGY

Plain Radiographs

In all cases of total hip replacement; anteroposterior (AP) pelvis radiographs, anteroposterior and lateral radiographs of both hips as well as AP radiographs of the femur are done. These should be correlated to the preoperative radiographs and immediate postoperative radiographs. In some cases, radiographs of the spine and knees should also be done. These radiographs may be normal even if there is some underlying pathology, therefore serial comparative films may be required. It is also a difficult task to differentiate between infection and loosening on plain radiographs (Figure 5).

Septic Loosening

Plain radiology does not reliably distinguish between septic and aseptic loosening. If loosening occurs early particularly in the first year or two and especially when there have been wound problems in the immediate postoperative period, septic loosening is considered more likely. In those cases, where we have a strong suspicion of infection you should look out for radiolucent lines (Figure 6) focal osteolysis with endosteal scalloping. In case, we observe any periosteal new bone formation then it is pathognomonic of infection and it is usually at metadiaphyseal junction on the medial side.

Aseptic Loosening

Criteria for aseptic loosening are different for both cemented and uncemented hips. It is easier to identify loosening in femur than acetabulum. The lucent lines don't necessarily represent problem, it may actually be present in well-fixed prosthesis also due to remodeling, etc.[33,34]

For Cemented Stems

• Subsidence
• Cement fracture
• Fractured stem
• Divergent or progressive radiolucency.

For Uncemented Stems

- Subsidence
- Distal pedestal formation (not simply a radiodense line at the tip of a cementless stem, but weight-bearing pedestal)
- Cortical hypertrophy
- Divergent radiolucency.

The defects have been classified by the American Academy of Orthopedic Surgeons (AAOS)[35-39] as follows:

- Segmental (cortical loss)
- Cavitary (contained lesion)
- Combined deficiencies
- Malalignment (rotational, angular)
- Femoral stenosis
- Femoral discontinuity.

Bone Scan

Tc99 Bone Scan: Bone scan are often nonspecific, and may show increased uptake in infection, loosening, heterotopic ossification, Paget's disease, stress fracture, large uncemented stem (modulus mismatch), tumors and reflex sympathetic dystrophy. The main advantage of a bone scan is that infective pathology is unlikely if it is negative. On the other hand, the disadvantage is that it is very sensitive, and has poor specificity as it doesn't differentiate between different causes of pain in the hip.[40] In cemented hips majority of scans would be normal by one year with 20% remain hot at some portions of stem, greater and lesser trochanter area. The uncemented hips can remain hot for 2 years and the distal stem for many more years.[41,42]

The other scan is the Indium-111 labeled leukocyte scan which is expensive and difficult because we have to harvest leukocytes. It is more specific for infection especially when combined with bone scan, having a sensitivity 92% and range specificity of 75 to 100%. In a study of patients suspected of having infected total hip replacements, FDG PET performed similarly to three-phase bone scintigraphy. FDG PET was more specific but less sensitive than conventional radiography for the diagnosis of infection.[43] RA and significant osteolysis are risk factor for false positive results.

MRI

MRI can also be a useful diagnostic tool in diagnosing the source of pain. It may pick-up some infective focus early on and help us in a culture biopsy of that particular region. It can also assess the soft tissue envelope as well as the prosthetic interface.[44]

ARTHROCENTESIS

Aspiration remains an essential part the diagnosis of an infected total joint, despite false negative rates of up to 15%. Aspiration cannot only confirm the diagnosis but also identify the offending organism, which guides antibiotic therapy. When the ESR and CRP are both elevated, the probability that a positive aspirate will confirm an infection is about 90%.[45]

The intraoperative frozen sections and gram stain are also very significant. The finding of acute inflammation, defined as 5 or more polymorphonuclear leu-

Infected prosthesis	All phases increased and usually diffuse in 3 phases
	Highly suggestive of infection
	Can get focal uptake similar to loosening but rarer
Loose prosthesis	Localized increased uptake on delayed phase only
	Motion of prosthesis causes increased bone turnover due to bone resorption
	Increased uptake at trochanters alone may be normal postoperative well advanced loosening can show diffuse uptake as for an infected hip change
Stress sites	Will see localized area of uptake on scan
	Corresponds with cortical thickening on plain X-rays
Insufficiency fracture	Occur in osteopenic patients
	Pubic rami fractures may cause groin pain
	Sacral fractures may cause posterior hip pain

Algorithm 1: Algorithm describing the approach to a case of painful THR

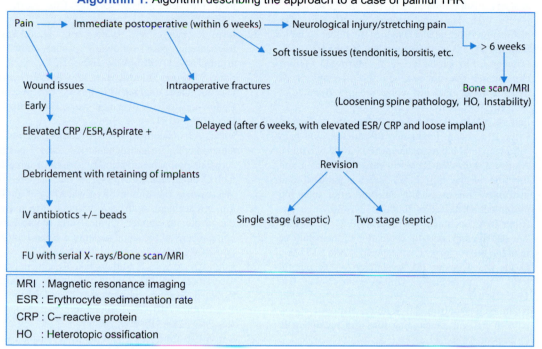

MRI : Magnetic resonance imaging
ESR : Erythrocyte sedimentation rate
CRP : C– reactive protein
HO : Heterotopic ossification

kocytes per high power field, has a high correlation with infection intraoperative frozen sections, and may be especially valuable at the time of reimplantation in the 2nd stage treatment of an infected prosthesis as a means to evaluate the sterility of the host bed.[46]

PCR: Polymerase chain reaction (PCR) analysis has been reported to have better specificity and sensitivity than standard culture methods. The technique involves the identification and amplification of the bacterial ribosomal RNA 16S fragment. A drawback of this technique is that it does not differentiate between live and dead bacteria and there may be a high number of false positive results.[47]

ALGORITHM (See Algorithm 1)

CONCLUSION

Postoperative pain after THA is often a diagnostic enigma if sufficient attention to detail is not paid. Causative factors in the early postoperative phase are different from the late presenting cases, and the surgeon has to focus on history, a detailed clinical examination and specific diagnostic modalities to obtain the correct diagnosis. An appropriate diagnosis allows adequate and timely management, which can often prevent deterioration of the joint.

REFERENCES

1. Hall MJ, Owings MF. 2000 National Hospital Discharge Survey. Hyattsville, MD: US Dept of Health and Human Services, Centers for Disease Control and Prevention, National Center for Health Statistics, 2002.

2. Pearl RE, et al. "Biomechanics and Pathomechanics of the Hip", The Art of THA by Grune and Stratton, Inc.

3. Paul JP. Load actions on the human femur during walking and some stress resultants, Exp Mech BR 1971;192:121-5.

4. Paul JP. Force actions transmitted by joints in the human body, Proc R Socv Lond (Bio) 1976; 192B:163-72.

5. Britton AR, Murray DW, Bulstrode CJ, McPherson K, Denham RA. Pain levels after total hip

replacement: their use as end points for survival analysis. J Bone Joint Surg Br 1997;79:93-8.

6. Harris WH. Traumatic arthritis of the hip after dislocation in acetabular fractures treatment by mold arthroplasty. J Bone Joint Surg Am 1969;51:737-55.

7. Dawson J, Fitzpatrick R, Carr A, Murray D. Oxford Hip Score: questionnaire on the perceptions of patients about total hip replacement. J Bone Joint Surg Br 1996;78:185-90.

8. Patrick J Duffy, Bassam A Masri, Donald S. Garbuz, Clive P. Duncan. Evaluation of patients with pain following total hip replacement JBJS 2005;87:A(11).

9. Alonso J, Lamarca R, Marti-Valls J. The pain and function of the hip (PFH) scale: a patient-based instrument for measuring outcome after total hip placement. Orthopedics 2000;23:1273-8.

10. Ritter MA, Fechtman RW, Keating EM, Faris PM. The use of a hip score for evaluation of the results of total hip arthroplasty. J Arthroplasty 1990;5:187-9.

11. Evans BG, Cuckler JM. Evaluation of the painful total hip arthroplasty. Orthop Clin North Am 1992;23:303.

12. Khan NQ, Woolson ST. Referral patterns of hip pain in patients undergoing total hip replacement. Orthopedics 1998;21:123.

13. Marmor L. Stress fracture of the pubic ramus stimulating a loose total hip replacement. Clin Orthop 1976;121:103.

14. Oh I, Hardacre JA. Fatigue fracture of the inferior pubic ramus following total hip replacement for congenital hip dislocation. Clin Orthop 1980; 147:154.

15. Siliski JM, Scott RD. Obturator-nerve palsy resulting from intrapelvic extrusion of cement during total hip replacement: report of four cases. J Bone Joint Surg Am 1985;67:1225.

16. Johanson NA, Pellicci PM, Tsairis P, Salvati EA. Nerve injury in total hip arthroplasty. Clin Orthop 1983;179:214.

17. Matos MH, Amstutz HC, Machleder HI: Ischemia of the lower extremity after total hip replacement. J Bone Joint Surg Am 1979;61:24.

18. Morrey BF, Adams RA, Cabanela ME: Comparison of heterotopic bone after anterolateral, transtrochanteric and posterior approaches for total hip arthroplasty. Clin Orthop 1984;188:160.

19. Bohl WR, Steffee AD. Lumbar spinal stenosis: a cause of continued pain and disability in patients after total hip arthroplasty. Spine 1979;4:168.

20. Floman Y, Bernini PM, Marvel JP Jr, Rothman RH. Low-back pain and sciatica following total hip replacement: a report of two cases. Spine 1980;5:292.

21. Evans BG, Cuckler JM. Evaluation of the painful total hip arthroplasty. Orthop Clin North Am 19992;23:303.

22. Iorio R, Healy WL, Warren PD, et al. Lateral trochanteric pain following primary total hip arthroplasty. J Arthroplasty 2006;21:233.

23. Saito S, Ryu J, Oikawa H, et al. Clinical results of Harris-Galante total hip arthroplasty without cement. Follow-up study of over five years. Bull Hosp Joint Dis 1997;56:191.

24. Vicar AJ, Coleman CR. A comparison of the anterolateral, transtrochanteric, and posterior surgical approaches in primary total hip arthroplasty. Clin Orthop Relat Res 1984;188:152.

25. Wiesman Jr HJ, Simon SR, Ewald FC, et al. Total hip replacement with and without osteotomy of the greater trochanter. Clinical and biomechanical comparisons in the same patients. J Bone Joint Surg Am 1978;60:203.

26. Engh CA, Massin P, Suthers KE. Roentgenographic assessment of the biologic fixation of porous-surfaced femoral components. Clin Orthop Relat Res 1990;257:107-28. Erratum in: Clin Orthop Relat Res. 1992;284:310-2.

27. Smith PN, Rorabeck CH. Clinical evaluation of the symptomatic total hip arthroplasty. In: Steinberg ME, Garino JP (Eds). Revision total hip arthroplasty. Philadelphia: Lippincott Williams and Wilkins;1999. pp. 109-120.

28. Johanson NA, Pellicci PM, Tsairis P, Salvati EA. Nerve injury in total hip arthroplasty. Clin Orthop Relat Res 1983;179:214-22.

29. Canner GC, Steinberg ME, Heppenstall RB, Balderston R. The infected hip after total hip arthroplasty. J Bone Joint Surg Am 1984;66:1393-9.

30. Aalto K, Osterman K, Peltola H, Rasanen J. Changes in erythrocyte sedimentation rate and C-reactive protein after total hip arthroplasty. Clin Orthop Relat Res 1984;184:118-20.

31. Sanzen L, Carlsson AS. The diagnostic value of C-reactive protein in infected total hip arthroplasties. J Bone Joint Surg Br 1989;71:638-41.

32. Spangehl MJ, Masri BA, O'Connell JX, Duncan CP. Prospective analysis of preoperative and intraoperative investigations for the diagnosis of infection at the sites of two hundred and two revision total hip arthroplasties. J Bone Joint Surg Am 1999;81:672-83.

33. O'Neill DA, Harris WH. Failed total hip replacement assessment by plain radiographs, arthrograms, and aspiration of the hip joint. J Bone Joint Surg Am 1984;66:540-6.

34. Jasty M, Maloney WJ, Bragdon CR, Haire T-Harris WH. Histomorphological studies of the long-term skeletal responses to well fixed cemented femoral components. J Bone Joint Surg Am 1990;72:1220-9.

35. Sinha RK, Shanbhag AS, Maloney WJ, Hasselman CT, Rubash HE. Osteolysis: Cause and Effect, Instructional Course Lectures, Volume 47. Rosemont, Ill: American Academy of Orthopedic Surgeons Press; 1998.pp.307-20.

36. Aseptic loosening in THA. In: American Academy of Orthopedic Surgeons. *Adult Reconstruction Orthopedic Knowledge Update.* Rosemont, Ill: American Academy of Orthopedic Surgeons Press; 1996./pp.147-56.

37. Berry DJ, Harmsen WS, Ilstrup DM. The natural history of debonding of the femoral component from the cement and its effect on long-term survival of Charnley total hip replacements. J Bone Joint Surg Am 1998;80:715-21.

38. D'Antonio JA, Capello WN, Borden LS, et al. Classification and management of acetabular abnormalities in total hip arthroplasty. Clin Orthop 1989;243:126-37.

39. Rubash HE, Sinha RK, Maloney WJ, Paprosky WG. Osteolysis: Surgical Treatment, Instructional Course Lectures, Volume 47. Rosemont, Ill: American Academy of Orthopedic Surgeons Press; 1998.pp. 321-9.

40. Lieberman JR, MH Huo, R Schneider, EA Salvati, S Rodi. Evaluation of painful hip arthroplasties. Are technetium bone scans necessary? Bone Joint Surg 1993;75B(3):475-8. Copyright © 1993 by British Editorial Society of Bone and Joint Surgery.

41. Ashbrooke, AB, Calvert PT. Bone scan appearances after uncemented hip replacement. J Royal Soc Med 1990;83:768-9.

42. Charito L, Maria BT, Scott EM, Paul VP, Christopher JP. Role of Nuclear Medicine in Diagnosis of the Infected Joint Replacement. Radio Graphics 2001;21: 1229-38.

43. Katrin DM Stumpe, Hubert P Nötzli, Marco Zanetti, Ehab M Kamel, Thomas F Hany, Gerhard W Görres, Gustav K von Schulthess, Juerg Hodler. FDG PET for Differentiation of Infection and Aseptic Loosening in Total Hip Replacements: comparison with conventional radiography and three-phase bone scintigraphy. Radiology 2004;231:333-41.

44. HJ Cooper, Ranawat AS, HG Potter, LF Foo, ST Jawetz, CS Ranawat. Magnetic Resonance Imaging in the Diagnosis and Management of Hip Pain After Total Hip Arthroplasty. The Journal of Arthroplasty 2009;24(5).

45. Spangehl MJ, Masri BA, O'Connell JX, et al. Prospective analysis of preoperative and intraoperative investigations for the diagnosis of infection at the sites of two hundred and two revision total hip arthroplasties. J Bone Joint Surg Am 1999; 81:672.

46. Mirra JM, Marder RA, Amstutz HC. The pathology of failed total join arthroplasty. Clin Orthop 1982; 170:175.

47. Mariani BD, Martin DS, Levine MJ, et al. The coventry award polymerase chain reaction detection of bacterial infection in total knee arthroplasty. Clin Orthop 1996;331:11.

EVALUATION OF PATIENTS WITH PAIN AFTER TOTAL HIP ARTHROPLASTY

Index